RADIOGRAPHIC PATHOLOGY WORKBOOK

RADIOGRAPHIC PATHOLOGY WORKBOOK

TerriAnn Linn-Watson, MEd, RT, RDMS
Associate Professor
Health Sciences Department
Chaffey College
Rancho Cucamonga, California

W.B. SAUNDERS COMPANY

A Division of Harcourt Brace & Company
Philadelphia London Toronto Montreal Sydney Tokyo

W.B. SAUNDERS COMPANY
A Division of Harcourt Brace & Company

The Curtis Center
Independence Square West
Philadelphia, Pennsylvania 19106

Library of Congress Cataloging-in-Publication Data

Radiographic Pathology Workbook

ISBN 0–7216–4169–5

Printed in United States of America

Last digit is the print number: 9   8   7   6   5   4   3   2

Preface

This workbook is designed to assist students of radiographic pathology in their efforts to learn about the sometimes complex disease processes that affect the different systems of the human. It is organized by chapters that correspond to the chapters in the textbook, *Radiographic Pathology*. The most effective method of learning is to complete each chapter of the workbook after reading each chapter of the textbook. Research in learning methods has proved that repeated exposure to important facts helps the student retain the information.

Each chapter begins with a rationale that helps students understand the relevance and application of the material covered in the chapter. Objectives are presented next. As the student masters each objective, he or she can check it off. This provides the student with a quick reference list of what competencies have been achieved. It further guides the student toward concentrating on unlearned areas. Quiz-type exercises are presented to reinforce understanding. Use of a variety of question formats helps the student comprehend the material and not simply memorize answers. The answers to the exercises are provided at the end of the workbook so that the student can determine in which areas he or she is weak and which areas he or she has mastered.

A self-test, similar to a final examination, is presented at the end of each chapter. This self-test should help determine if all objectives have been met and competency has been achieved. This learning method challenges students to do much of the critical thinking on their own. A scoring standard has been set at 94%. This high percentage challenges the student to perform at an exceptional level. These are the students who will become radiographers who are the top performers in the field and be indispensable to an imaging department that runs on the creative abilities of its technologists.

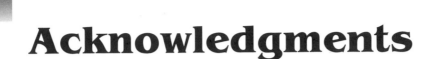

Acknowledgments

I am pleased to acknowledge and recognize those persons who have provided support and encouragement during the preparation of this student workbook.

The graduating class of 1995 from Chaffey College's Radiologic Technology Program had the "opportunity" to take each of the self-tests as homework assignments. Without their invaluable arguments, many of the questions would have remained vague or incomplete. My biggest thanks goes to all of them!

My colleague, Andrea Guillen-Dutton, RT (R,M), carried many of the professional duties that I had previously undertaken so that I could meet deadlines. Besides the much-needed time-outs with flavored coffees and a shopping spree, she allowed me to rant, rave, and sometimes throw tantrums, yet never held it against me.

I would be remiss if I did not say thank-you to Ellen Thomas, who sent every page of my original work back to me for my okay before sending the material into production. Thank you, Ellen.

Finally, but most important to me, are the acknowledgments and thanks to my sons, Kendrick and Kamden, for their tremendous maturity at such tender ages. You both understood me and the pressures far more than most adults. I love both of you.

talw

Contents

Speciality x 30
Midterm x 15
Cards x 10

Pathology x 30
final x 15

Introduction

This workbook should be completed as each chapter of the textbook is read. It has been proved by research in learning methods that repeated exposure to important facts helps the student retain the information.

When this workbook is used in conjunction with the textbook, learning is combined into a logical sequence. The following advantages are provided with this student workbook:

1. A rationale precedes each chapter to help the student understand the relevance and application of the material covered in the chapter.

2. Objectives presented at the beginning of each chapter can be checked off as each is mastered, thus guiding the student toward concentration on unlearned areas.

3. Each chapter emphasizes only material that is important to the radiographer.

4. The material is presented in a logical sequence. Quiz-type exercises are presented to reinforce understanding. Answers are provided so that the student can determine which areas are weak and which have been mastered.

A self-test, similar to a final examination, is presented at the end of each chapter. This self-test should help determine if all objectives have been mastered and competency has been achieved.

This learning method challenges students to do much of the critical thinking on their own. Remember, mastery comes with repetition.

Student Instructions

You should read the introduction, which will help you understand the learning method presented in this workbook. It will help you understand the importance of completing each area and reviewing those areas not fully mastered.

You should read the rationale preceding each chapter so that you understand why you need to learn this material and how you will use it. Check off the objectives as they are successfully completed. Those objectives that remain unchecked serve as a study guide for review of the material needing mastery. Once you have completed all exercises and checked off all objectives, you are ready for the self-test, which should help you determine if you have not only learned the material, but also retained it. You should take the self-test in a regular test situation. All questions asked in the self-test can be found in the exercises. When you have completed the self-test, check your answers with those found in the exercises. A score of 80 to 89 percent indicates you have an understanding of the material; however, you should review the points you have missed. A score of 90 percent indicates you have mastered the material and are ready to move on. Scores of 95 percent and higher are demonstrative of comprehension and retention at a high level. You should be able to complete evaluations based on the objectives of the workbook and textbook with high scores.

Pathology
Principles

Rationale

An understanding of basic principles of pathology and an awareness of the radiographic appearance of specific diseases are essential parts of the training of a radiologic technologist. A technologist is aided in the selection of proper modalities and in determining the need for a repeat radiograph when disease processes are properly understood. Many types of diseases exist, and many conditions can be demonstrated radiographically. The role of the radiologic technologist is to display visually the changes in normal anatomy and tissue density caused by disease.

When the radiographer can reasonably determine a patient's disease process by the manifestations observed, radiographic positioning and technique are modified to compensate for the specific pathology, thus eliminating repeat radiographs.

Objectives

1. Define the following terms:

( ) pathology	( ) etiology
( ) disease process	( ) morbidity rate
( ) pathogenesis	( ) mortality rate
( ) diagnosis	( ) idiopathic
( ) prognosis	( ) phagocytosis
( ) procedures	( ) metaplasia
( ) test	( ) infarct
( ) manifestation	( ) iatrogenic
( ) symptom	( ) ischemia
( ) sign	( ) congestion
( ) history	( ) atrophy
( ) syndrome	( ) necrosis
( ) frequency	( ) hypoxia
( ) incidence	( ) exudate
( ) hyperplasia	( ) hypoplasia
( ) hypertrophy	( ) transudate

2. ( ) Define structural disease.

3. ( ) Define functional disease.

4. ( ) List two examples of structural diseases.

5. ( ) List one example of functional disease.

6. ( ) Describe acute injury.

7. ( ) List one example of acute injury.

8. ( ) Describe chronic injury.

9. ( ) List two examples of chronic injury.

10. ( ) List and describe four types of atrophy.

11. ( ) Explain the difference between thrombus and embolus.

12. ( ) List the five signs of acute inflammation.

13. ( ) Describe the two types of body repair mechanism.

14. ( ) List the fundamental tissues.

15. ( ) Define growth disturbances.

16. ( ) List two examples of benign and malignant growth disturbances.

17. ( ) Describe the difference between hyperplasia and neoplasm.

18. ( ) List the ways cancer spreads.

19. ( ) Define grading of a tumor.

20. ( ) Define staging of a tumor.

EXERCISE I-1

Complete the blanks in the following statements.

1. A disease is a morbid process usually having

   specific ___Symptoms___ and, sometimes,

   physical ___signs___ .

2. Factors to be considered in making a diagnosis include evaluations of the

   patient known as a ___procedure___ and analysis of

   specimens known as a ___test___ .

3. Physical and/or biochemical changes within a cell are

called ___lesions___ .

4. Clinical ___manifestation___ may point to a diagnosis. If not, the patient may have a radiographic examination. These examinations

are known as ___procedures___ .

5. The ratio of actual deaths to expected deaths is known as

the ___mortality___ rate.

6. Sublethal cell injury is also known

as ___degeneration___ .

7. Direct physical injury by an object is

called ___trauma___ .

8. The leading internal cause of structural disease

is ___P vascular___ disease.

9. List the four cardinal signs of inflammation.

___red skin___   ___swelling___

___heat___   ___pain___

10. Name the sequence of events which occurs in inflammation.

___alteration in vascularity___   ___phagocytosis___

___leukocytes go to area___   ___repair___

11. Name the four types of fundamental tissue.

Epithelial   _connective_

muscle   _Nervous_

12. What are the three types of muscle cells?

voluntary   _cardiac_

involuntary

13. The two types of primary repair that the body will attempt

are _regeneration_

and _Granulation_ .

14. The two categories of growth disturbances

are _neoplasms_

and _hyper plasia_ .

EXERCISE I-2

Mark the following statements "T" for true or "F" for false. If it is a false statement, reword it to make it true by changing the incorrect portions.

_T_   1. Disease may affect only one organ primarily but also affect another organ secondarily.

_F_   2. A barium enema is a ~~test.~~ _procedure_

_T_   3. The function of an organ may be impaired yet there may be no structural defects.

_T_   4. Arrhythmia (irregular heart beat) is a sign.

_F_   _functional_
5. Two classifications of disease are structural and ~~organic.~~

_F_   _structural_
6. An allergic disease is a ~~functional~~ disease.

_T_   7. Radiation is an example of a physical disease-causing agent.

_T_   8. The leading cause of death resulting from vascular insufficiency is a myocardial infarct. (heart attack)

_F_   _blood_
9. Congestion is due to ~~exudate~~ filling up the pleural cavity.

_F_   _least_
10. Granulation tissue repair is ~~most~~ desirable.

_T_   11. Nervous cell tissue is the most specialized in the body.

_F_   _Epithelial_
12. ~~Connective~~ tissue serves as a lining for body spaces.

_T_   13. Transudate is serum fluid that passes through a membrane.

_F_   _external_
14. Physical and chemical substances are examples of ~~internal~~ disease-causing agents.

_F_   15. An analysis performed on a specimen removed from a patient is known as a ~~procedure.~~ test.

EXERCISE 1-3

Circle the letter in front of the correct answer.

_A_ 1. An example of a procedure is a(n)
    A. arthrogram
    B. CBC
    C. UA
    D. biopsy of a frozen section

_C_ 2. A headache is an example of a
    A. syndrome
    B. sign
    C. symptom
    D. manifestation

_B_ 3. Ratio of sick to well persons in a given area is called the
    A. mortality rate
    B. morbidity rate
    C. prevalence
    D. frequency

A 4.   Which is *not* in the structural disease category?
    A.   pathophysiologic changes
    B.   genetic diseases
    C.   acquired injuries
    D.   hyperplasias

D 5.   Which are examples of internal mechanisms for injury?
    (1) vascular insufficiency   (2) immunologic reactions   (3) metabolic disturbances
    A.   1 and 2
    B.   1 and 3
    C.   2 and 3
    D.   1, 2, and 3

D 6.   External causes of disease are
    (1) physical   (2) chemical   (3) microbiologic
    A.   1 and 2
    B.   1 and 3
    C.   2 and 3
    D.   1, 2, and 3

A 7.   Memory impairment occurs with which type of atrophy?
    A.   senile
    B.   disuse
    C.   pressure
    D.   endocrine

A 8.   Which are examples of chronic inflammation?
    (1) asthma   (2) hayfever   (3) peritonitis
    A.   1 and 2
    B.   1 and 3
    C.   2 and 3
    D.   1, 2, and 3

B 9.   Pus filling the pleural cavity is known as
    A.   abscess
    B.   empyema
    C.   purulent exudate
    D.   suppurative inflammation

C 10.   The most widespread tissue of the body is
    A.   nervous cell tissue
    B.   muscle cell tissue
    C.   connective tissue
    D.   epithelial tissue

A 11.   The relationship between the occurrence of disease and the reproductive capability of the cell is
    A.   direct
    B.   indirect
    C.   has no bearing
    D.   dependent on the disease

_C_ 12. The spread of malignant tumor cells to a distant site is known as
   A. carcinogenesis
   B. hyperplasia
   C. metastasis
   D. contagious

_A_ 13. If the condition existed at or before birth, it is said to be
   A. congenital
   B. chronic
   C. hereditary
   D. atypical

EXERCISE I-4

Match each of the following with the correct definition by placing the letter of the answer in the space provided. Each question has only one correct answer.

A. etiology	L. ischemia	W. test
B. manifestations	M. congestion	X. mortality rate
C. idiopathic	N. prognosis	Y. repair
D. nosocomial	O. atrophy	Z. prevalence
E. anoxia	P. growth disturbance	AA. transudate
F. phagocytosis	Q. necrosis	BB. hyperplasia
G. metaplasia	R. hypoxia	CC. thrombus
H. pathogenesis	S. dysplasia	DD. incidence
I. infarct	T. exudate	EE. pathology
J. iatrogenic	U. embolus	FF. hypertrophy
K. disease process	V. diagnosis	GG. frequency

1. __Y__ body's attempt to return to normal *repair*

2. __P__ any type of lesion or tissue mass characterized by the reproductive capability of the cell *growth disturbance*

3. __N__ predicted course of a disease and the prospects for recovery *prognosis*

4. __S__ abnormal development of tissue characterized by loss of normal uniformity of individual cells *dysplasia*

5. __G__ cell changing from normal to abnormal *metaplasia*

6. __U__ a traveling thrombus *embolus*

7. _O_ progressive wasting away of any part of the body resulting in impaired function or loss of function *atrophy*

8. _M_ capillary filling *congesting*

9. _F_ digestion of bacteria by leukocytes *phagocytosis*

10. _AA_ clear serum fluid that passes through a membrane or tissue *transudate*

11. _T_ thick, cloudy fluid that passes through a membrane or tissue *exudate*

12. _C_ diseases of unknown causes *idiopathic*

13. _J_ adverse reactions while under the care of a physician *iatrogenic*

14. _D_ that which was acquired from a hospital environment *nosocomial*

15. _Q_ death of cells *necrosis*

16. _E_ lack of oxygen *anoxia*

17. _R_ reduced oxygen *hypoxia*

18. _CC_ mass (blood clots) adhering to a vessel wall *thrombus*

19. _EE_ study of disease *pathology*

20. _A_ study of the cause of disease *etiology*

21. _H_ sequence of events that renders the disease apparent *pathogenesis*

22. _B_ observed changes due to disease *manifestation*

23. _L_ deficiency of blood in the muscle *ischemia*

24. _I_ area of dead or necrotic tissue *infarct*

25. _W_ analysis of specimens taken from a patient *test*

26. _K_ abnormal change that takes place in the body *disease process*

27. _FF_ increase in cell size *hypertrophy*

28. _BB_ increase in cell number *hyperplasia*

29. _Z_ number of people with a disease at any point in time *prevalence*

30. _GG_ rate of occurrence measured over a given period of time *frequency*

31. _V_ the determination of what disease a person has *diagnosis*

32. _DD_ number of newly diagnosed causes of a disease in 1 year *incidence*

33. _X_ ratio of actual deaths to expected deaths *mortality rate*

CHAPTER I SELF-TEST

There are 50 possible points on this self-test. Score it against the answers found in the exercises. A score of 47 points or higher indicates mastery and retention of this material.

Complete the blanks in the following statements.

1. Leading internal cause of structural disease

   is ___*Vascular*___ disease.

2. Name the four types of fundamental tissue:

   ___*epithual*___   ___*Nervous*___

   ___*connective*___   ___*muscle*___

3. The two categories of growth disturbances

   are ___*neoplasm*___

   and ___*hyperplasia*___ .

4. What are the three types of muscle cells?

   ___*voluntary*___   ___*cardiac*___

   ___*involuntary*___

5. List the four cardinal signs of inflammation.

   ___*red skin*___   ___*heat*___

   ___*swelling*___   ___*pain*___

6. The two types of primary repair that the body will attempt

   are ___*regeneration*___

   and ___*granulation tissue*___.

7. Physical and/or biochemical changes within a cell are

called *lesions* .

8. The ratio of actual deaths to expected deaths is known as

the *Mortality* rate.

9. Sublethal cell injury is also known

as *degeneration* .

Match each of the following with the correct definition by placing the letter of the answer in the space provided. Each question has only one correct answer.

A. prognosis

B. pathogenesis

C. manifestations

D. phagocytosis

E. pathology

F. nosocomial

G. frequency

H. anoxia

I. ischemia

J. idiopathic

K. disease process

L. mortality rate

M. dysplasia

N. congestion

O. transudate

P. atrophy

Q. etiology

R. exudate

S. infarct

T. incidence

10. __A__ predicted course of a disease and the prospects for recovery

11. __M__ abnormal development of tissue characterized by loss of normal uniformity of individual cells

12. __P__ progressive wasting away of any part of the body resulting in impaired function or loss of function

13. __N__ capillary filling

14. __D__ digestion of bacteria by leukocytes

15. __O__ clear serum fluid that passes through a membrane or tissue

16. __R__ thick, cloudy fluid that passes through a membrane or tissue

17. __J__ diseases of unknown causes

18. __F__ that which was acquired from a hospital environment

19. __H__ lack of oxygen

20. __E__ study of disease

21. __Q__ study of the cause of disease

22. __B__ sequence of events that renders the disease apparent

23. __C__ observed changes due to disease

24. _I_ deficiency of blood in the muscle

25. _S_ area of dead or necrotic tissue

26. _K_ abnormal change that takes place in the body

27. _G_ rate of occurrence measured over a given period of time

28. _T_ number of newly diagnosed cases of a disease in 1 year

29. _L_ ratio of actual deaths to expected deaths

Mark the following statements "T" for true or "F" for false.

_F_ 30. ~~Connective~~ Epithial tissue serves as a lining for body spaces.

_F_ 31. A barium enema is a ~~test.~~ proccedure

_F_ 32. Two classifications of disease are structural and ~~organic.~~ functional

_T_ 33. Radiation is an example of a physical disease-causing agent.

_T_ 34. Transudate is serum fluid that passes through a membrane.

_F_ 35. Congestion is due to ~~exudate~~ increase blood in capillaries filling up the pleural cavity.

_F_ 36. Physical and chemical substances are examples of ~~internal~~ external disease-causing agents.

_T_ 37. Disease may affect only one organ primarily but may also affect another organ secondarily.

_T_ 38. The function of an organ may be impaired yet there may be no structural defects.

_T_ 39. Arrhythmia (irregular heart beat) is a sign.

_T_ 40. The leading cause of death resulting from vascular insufficiency is a myocardial infarct.

Circle the letter in front of the correct answer.

_A_ 41. Which is not a structural disease category?
   A. pathophysiologic changes
   B. genetic diseases
   C. acquired injuries
   D. hyperplasias

_C_ 42. The spread of malignant tumor cells to a distant site is
   A. carcinogenesis
   B. hyperplasia
   C. metastasis
   D. contagious

_C_ 43. The most widespread tissue of the body is
   A. nervous cell tissue
   B. muscle cell tissue
   C. connective tissue
   D. epithelial tissue

_A_ 44. Which are examples of chronic inflammation?
   (1) asthma   (2) hayfever   (3) peritonitis
   A. 1 and 2 only
   B. 1 and 3 only
   C. 2 and 3 only
   D. 1, 2, and 3

_A_ 45. If the condition existed at or before birth, it is said to be
   A. congenital
   B. chronic
   C. hereditary
   D. atypical

_A_ 46. An example of a procedure is a(n)
   A. arthrogram
   B. CBC
   C. UA
   D. biopsy of a frozen section

_D_ 47. External causes of disease are
   (1) physical   (2) chemical   (3) microbiologic
   A. 1 and 2
   B. 1 and 3
   C. 2 and 3
   D. 1, 2, and 3

_C_ 48. A headache is an example of a
   A. syndrome
   B. sign
   C. symptom
   D. manifestation

_A_ 49. The relationship between the occurrence of disease and the reproductive capa-
   bility of the cell
   A. is direct
   B. is indirect
   C. has no bearing
   D. is dependent on the disease

_B_ 50. Ratio of sick to well persons in a given area is called the
A. mortality rate
B. morbidity rate
C. prevalence
D. frequency

Contrast Media

Rationale

Approximately 30 percent of all radiologic examinations involve the use of some form of contrast media to aid in the visualization of a body part or a body system. Thus, one must have at least a fundamental knowledge of contrast media. The technologist must be able to evaluate the patient's chart and determine the effect contrast agents will have in light of specific laboratory results. It is extremely important for the radiographer to be able to anticipate and recognize adverse reactions the patient may experience from the injection of contrast media. Because these may be life-threatening to the patient, a quick response is essential. Even the routine urogram can quickly become serious in the event a patient experiences a reaction and the technologist is not able to respond.

Objectives

1. ( ) Name the three classifications of contrast agents.

2. ( ) List the four types of radiolucent contrast agents.

3. ( ) List the characteristics of radiolucent contrast.

4. ( ) List the characteristics of radiopaque contrast.

5. ( ) Describe the composition of radiopaque contrast.

6. ( ) Define ionic contrast.

7. ( ) Define nonionic contrast.

8. ( ) Compare the composition of ionic and nonionic contrasts.

9. ( ) Explain the difference between cholecystographics and cholecystogogues.

10. ( ) Name the three classifications of adverse reactions.

11. ( ) List the minor reactions.

12. ( ) Name the drugs given for urticaria.

13. ( ) Explain the types of respiratory distress encountered with an intermediate reaction.

14. ( ) Explain what happens during a major reaction.

15. ( ) Define vasovagal reactions.

16. Explain each of the following conditions for contrast selection.

( ) Toxicity   ( ) Iodine content
( ) Miscibility   ( ) Osmolality
( ) Persistence   ( ) Ionic Salt
( ) Viscosity

17. List the contrast used in each system.

( ) Biliary   ( ) Genitourinary
( ) Gastrointestinal ( ) Neurogenic
( ) Salivary ducts   ( ) Respiratory
( ) Reproductive   ( ) Lymph system

EXERCISE II-1

Complete the blanks in the following statements.

1. A reaction due to fear of the examination is known as

   a _Vasovagal_ reaction.

2. When an intermediate reaction to contrast occurs, what drug is given

   first? _Benedryl_

3. Name the four negative contrast agents that are used.

   Oxygen   _nitrous Oxide_

   carbon dioxide   _air_

4. What two negative contrast agents are dangerous?

   Oxygen   _air_

5. Two negative contrast agents can be dangerous because they can cause

   a _gas_   _emboli_ .

6. Name the only inert contrast agent. _barium_

7. Name the three reasons iodine is used in soluble contrast materials.

availibility   _exchangbility w/ other_
atomic number   _ions_

8. Use of a positive contrast media (increases, decreases)

increases _____ the organ density by using

a substance with a (high, low) _high_ _____
atomic number.

9. Negative contrast agents use a substance with a (high, low)

low _____ atomic weight to (increase, decrease)

decrease _____ the density of the organ.

10. What must be obtained before injecting a patient with a contrast agent?

allergic   _history_

11. In x-ray, contrast means _density_ _____ difference.

12. A patient who is flushed and has nausea is probably having a

minor _____ reaction.

13. What laboratory value should be checked before an IVP?

Bun _____ Before a gallbladder examination?

Bilirubin

14. Name the four major groups of positive contrast media by their chemical structure.

    nonionic _____ monomers;

    ionic _____ monomers;

    ionic _monoacid_ _____ dimers;

    nonionic _____ dimers.

15. Ionic monomers have ____ _3_ _____ iodine atoms

    and _____ _2_ _____ particles in solution
    for osmolality.

16. What chemical compound is eliminated and replaced with a hydroxyl group to obtain low osmolality contrast media?

    Carboxyl _____ group

17. Name the seven characteristics which should be addressed before choosing a contrast media.

    Viscosity _____   _persistance_ _____

    miscibility _____   _type of ionic salt_ _____

    toxicity _____   _ionic content_ _____

    osmality _____

18. How much iodine concentration is needed for adequate opacity on

    radiographs? ____ _300_ _____ mg/mL

EXERCISE II-2

Mark the following statements "T" for true or "F" for false. If it is a false statement, reword it to make it true by changing the incorrect portion(s).

_T_ 1. Contrast agents are pharmaceuticals.

_T_ 2. Radiolucents decrease organ density.

_F_ 3. ~~Ultrasonography~~ *Nuclear med* uses radionuclides.

_T_ 4. Air as a contrast agent can cause an embolus.

→ _F_ 5. Radiopaques are also called ~~negative~~ *positive* contrast agents.

→ _T_ 6. All soluble positive contrast media contain some form of iodine.

→ _T_ 7. A characteristic of radionuclides is the emission of radiation.

_T_ 8. Iodine is easily exchangeable with other ions.

_F_ 9. All positive contrast agents are ~~absorbed by the body~~ *excreted by liver or kidney*.

→ _T_ 10. Viscosity is a factor to consider when choosing a contrast agent.

_F_ 11. If a contrast agent has high toxicity, it is ~~good~~ *not* to use.

_F_ 12. Ethiodol has ~~high~~ *low* miscibility. *oily / doesn't mix*

→ _T_ 13. Ultimately the choice of a contrast agent is left to the radiologist.

→ _F_ 14. ~~Dionosil~~ *Tekpaque* is used for gallbladder examinations.

_T_ 15. Hypaque causes dehydration.

→ _T_ 16. Fear of the examination can cause a vasovagal reaction.

→ _F_ 17. An adverse reaction is sure to occur when injecting meglumine diatrizoate ~~slowly~~ *fast*.

_F_ 18. Solu-Cortef is given for ~~minor reactions~~ *cardiac arrest*.

_T_ 19. Always take an allergic history.

_T_ 20. Most iodinated contrast materials are excreted unchanged by either the liver or the kidney.

_F_ ~~Negative~~ *positive* contrast agents are made up of an anion and a cation.

_F_ 22. The more meglumine salt, the ~~higher~~ *lower* the iodine content that is delivered to the body per second during injection.

_T_ 23. As iodine content rises, so does the viscosity of the contrast agent.

_T_ 24. Meglumine salt compounds are more viscous than sodium salt compounds; therefore, they have more iodine than sodium salt compounds.

_F_ 25. When a fistula exists between the bowel and peritoneum, ~~Gastrografin should~~ never be used to study the bowel.
Never use barium

_T_ 26. Positive contrast media have a high atomic weight.

_T_ 27. Radionuclides are a form of contrast media.

_T_ 28. Ionic and nonionic compounds contain iodine.

EXERCISE II-3

Circle the letter in front of the correct answer.

1. Which of the following is *not* a contrast agent used for the biliary system?
   A. Telepaque
   B. Amipaque
   C. Oragrafin
   D. Cholografin

2. Which of the following is a characteristic of a radiopaque agent?
   A. low atomic weight
   B. increases film density
   C. relatively nontoxic
   D. decreases organ density

3. Which is not a classification of contrast agents?
   A. radionuclides
   B. radiopaques
   C. radiolucents
   D. radiointensifiers

4. When choosing a contrast agent, which characteristic is *not* wanted?
   A. low osmolality
   B. high miscibility
   C. high toxicity
   D. high persistence

5. A patient who is flushed and has nausea and vomiting but no other symptoms is experiencing what type of reaction?
   A. vasovagal
   B. mild
   C. intermediate
   D. major

6. Possible adverse reactions to intravascularly injected iodinated contrast media include
   (1) urticaria   (2) dyspnea   (3) hypotension
   A. 1 and 2
   B. 1 and 3
   C. 2 and 3
   D. 1, 2, and 3

7. Which of the following statements regarding the use of radiographic contrast agents is *false?*
   A. atomic number is a factor in the choice of an agent
   B. rapid absorption or excretion by the body is advantageous
   C. similar density to the radiographed organ enhances contrast
   D. hollow organs require the use of contrast media

8. Contrast media are used to
   A. improve image sharpness
   B. improve radiographic latitude
   C. increase tissue contrast
   D. decrease tissue opacity

9. Iodine is used in soluble contrast materials for all of the following reasons except
   A. its availability
   B. its atomic number
   C. its exchangeability with other ions
   D. its amount of diatrizoate salts

10. As iodine content of the contrast agent rises, the viscosity
    A. rises
    B. falls
    C. remains the same
    D. goes either way depending on the miscibility of the agent

11. High tonicity of contrast agents causes
    (1) reduced contrast owing to dilution   (2) electrolytes to be drawn into bowel   (3) water to be hypersecreted from the kidneys
    A. 1 and 2
    B. 1 and 3
    C. 2 and 3
    D. 1, 2, and 3

12. Which is *not* an example of an ionic monomer?
    A. Renografin
    B. Hypaque
    C. Conray
    D. Isovue

13. Which term refers to osmolality equal to body fluids?
    A. iso-osmolar
    B. hyperosmolar
    C. hypo-osmolar
    D. osmophilic

14. Which are the most commonly used ionic salts?
    (1) sodium   (2) carbonate   (3) meglumine
    A. 1 and 2
    B. 1 and 3
    C. 2 and 3
    D. 1, 2, and 3

EXERCISE II-4

Match the following by placing the letter of the answer in the space provided.

A. radiopaque

B. radiolucent

1. __A__ high atomic weight

2. __B__ absorbed by the body

3. __B__ decreased absorption of x-ray

4. __A__ decreased film density

5. __B__ decreased organ density

6. __B__ negative contrast

7. __B__ low atomic weight

8. __A__ relatively nontoxic

9. __A__ absorbs more radiation

10. __A__ readily excreted by the kidneys

11. __B__ increases film density

12. __A__ increases organ density

EXERCISE II-5

For the systems listed in Table II–1, mark an "X" by those contrast media that can be used to demonstrate each particular system.

Table II–1.

Examinations of Systems

	Biliary	Gastrointestinal	Respiratory	Urinary	Reproductive	Neurogenic
Salpix					X	
Hypaque	X	X		X		
Gastrografin		X				
Cholografin	X					
Isovue	X			X		X
Conray	X			X		
Renografin	X			X		
Telepaque	X					
Lipiodol					X	
Oragrafin	X					
Sinografin					X	
Ethiodol					X	
Omnipaque				X	X	X
Dionosil			X			

CHAPTER II SELF-TEST

There are 50 possible points on this self-test. Score it against the answers found in the exercises. A score of 47 points or higher indicates mastery and retention of this material.

Complete the blanks in the following statements.

1. Use of a positive contrast medium _increase_ the organ density by using a substance with

   a _high_ atomic weight.

2. In radiography, contrast means _density_ difference.

3. Ionic monomers contain _____3_____ iodine

atoms and _____2_____ particles in solution for osmolality.

4. When an intermediate reaction to a contrast agent occurs, what drug is given

first? _Benedryl_

5. Negative contrast agents use a substance with

a _low_ atomic weight

to _decrease_ the density of the organ.

→ 6. What laboratory value should be checked before an

IVP? _Bun_ Before a gallbladder

examination? _Serum bilirubin_

7. What must be obtained before injecting a patient with a contrast

agent? _history_

8. Name the four major groups of positive contrast media by their chemical structure.

nonionic monomers;

ionic monomers;

ionic _nonionic_ dimers;

ionic dimers

→ 9. Name the only inert contrast agent. _barium_

10. A patient who is flushed and has nausea is probably having

a _____*mild*_____ reaction.

11. Name the four negative contrast agents that are used.

_____*nitrous acid*_____   _____*air*_____

_____*oxygen*_____   _____*carbon dioxide*_____

12. What two negative contrast agents are dangerous?

_____*air*_____   _____*oxygen*_____

Mark the following statements "T" for true or "F" for false.

_T___ 13. Most iodinated contrast materials are excreted unchanged by either the liver or the kidney.

_F___ *Radioluscents* 14. ~~Radiopaques~~ are also called negative contrast agents.

_T___ 15. A characteristic of radionuclides is that they emit radiation.

_F___ 16. Solu-Cortef is given for *cardiac* ~~minor~~ reactions.

_F___ 17. All positive contrast agents are *excreted* ~~absorbed~~ by the body.

_F___ *Telepaque* 18. ~~Dionosil~~ is used for gallbladder examinations.

_T___ 19. Contrast agents are pharmaceuticals.

_F___ *NUC MED* ← 20. ~~Ultrasonography~~ uses radionuclides.

_T___ 21. Positive contrast media have a high atomic weight.

_T___ 22. Fear of the examination can cause a vasovagal reaction.

_T___ 23. Viscosity is a factor to consider when choosing a media.

_F___ 24. The more meglumine salt, the *lower* ~~higher~~ the iodine content that is delivered to the body per second during injection.

_F_ ____ 25. When a fistula exists between the bowel and peritoneum, Gastrografin should never be used to study the bowel.

_f_ ____ 26. ~~Negative~~ Positive contrast agents are made up of an anion and a cation.

_T_ ____ 27. All soluble positive contrast media contain some form of iodine.

_T_ ____ 28. Always take an allergic history.

_T_ ____ 29. Ionic and nonionic compounds contain iodine.

_T_ ____ 30. Meglumine salt compounds are more viscous than sodium salt compounds; therefore, they have more iodine than sodium salt compounds.

_T_ ____ 31. Iodine is easily exchangeable with other ions.

_T_ ____ 32. Hypaque causes dehydration.

Circle the letter in front of the correct answer.

33. Which of the following is *not* a contrast agent used for the biliary system?
    A. Telepaque
    B. Amipaque
    C. Oragrafin
    D. Cholografin

34. Which is *not* a classification of contrast agents?
    A. radionuclides
    B. radiopaques
    C. radiolucents
    D. radiointensifiers

35. A patient who is flushed and has nausea and vomiting but no other symptoms is experiencing what type of reaction?
    A. vasovagal
    B. mild
    C. intermediate
    D. major

36. Which of the following statements regarding the use of radiographic contrast agents is *false?*
    A. atomic number is a factor in the choice of an agent
    B. rapid absorption or excretion by the body is advantageous
    C. similar density to the radiographed organ enhances contrast
    D. hollow organs require the use of contrast media

37. High tonicity of contrast agents causes
    (1) reduced contrast owing to dilution (2) electrolytes to be drawn into bowel (3) water to be hypersecreted from the kidneys
    A. 1 and 2
    B. 1 and 3
    C. 2 and 3
    D. 1, 2, and 3

38. Which term refers to osmolality equal to body fluids?
    A. iso-osmolar
    B. hyperosmolar
    C. hypo-osmolar
    D. osmophilic

39. Iodine is used in soluble contrast materials for all of the following reasons *except*
    A. its availability
    B. its atomic number
    C. its exchangeability with other ions
    D. its amount of diatrizoate salts

40. Which of the following is a characteristic of a radiopaque agent?
    A. low atomic weight
    B. increases film density
    C. relatively nontoxic
    D. decreases organ density

41. When choosing a contrast agent, which characteristic is *not* wanted?
    A. low osmolality
    B. high miscibility
    C. high toxicity
    D. high persistence

42. Possible adverse reactions to intravascularly injected iodinated contrast media include
    (1) urticaria   (2) dyspnea   (3) hypotension
    A. 1 and 2
    B. 1 and 3
    C. 2 and 3
    D. 1, 2, and 3

43. As iodine content of the contrast agent rises, the viscosity
    A. rises
    B. falls
    C. remains the same
    D. goes either way depending on the miscibility of the agent

44. Contrast media are used to
    A. improve image sharpness
    B. improve radiographic latitude
    C. increase tissue contrast
    D. decrease tissue opacity

Match the following by placing the letter of the answer in the space provided.

A. radiopaque

B. radiolucent

45. _A_ high atomic weight

46. _B_ decreased absorption of x-ray

47. _A_ decreased film density

48. _B_ low atomic weight

49. _A_ absorbs more radiation

50. _B_ absorbed by the body

Skeletal System

Rationale

Many of the patients that are seen in the radiography department have been involved in a traumatic injury causing discomfort or pain. The technologist must be aware of what the patient is experiencing in order to prevent any further complications. An understanding of the pathologic processes involved in the different nonneoplastic and neoplastic bone diseases helps prevent unnecessary repeat radiographs owing to inappropriate technical factors.

Objectives

1. (   ) Name the two classifications of the skeleton.

2. (   ) List the five types of bones and give examples of each.

3. (   ) Define the three types of joints in the body.

4. (   ) Describe the process of ossification.

5. (   ) Explain how bones grow in length and diameter.

6. (   ) List the functions of the skeletal system.

7. (   ) Describe an arthrogram procedure.

8. (   ) Describe the different types of transitional vertebrae.

9. (   ) Explain sacralization.

10. (   ) Compare and contrast osteoporosis and osteomalacia.

11. (   ) Describe achondroplasia.

12. (   ) Define rickets.

13. (   ) Describe the radiographic appearance of renal osteodystrophy.

14. (   ) Explain the process of osteomyelitis.

15. (   ) Explain how acromegaly relates to Paget disease.

16. (   ) Define the radiographic appearance of Legg-Calvé-Perthes disease.

17. (   ) List three types of chondromas.

18. (   ) Describe the appearance of osteochondroma.

19. (   )   Name the four chief primary malignant bone tumors.

20. (   )   Explain the process of how a fracture heals.

21. Define the following fracture terms:

( ) simple   ( ) comminuted   ( ) impacted
( ) complete   ( ) reduced   ( ) compression
( ) fissure   ( ) displacement   ( ) plastic
( ) closed   ( ) distraction   ( ) greenstick
( ) compound   ( ) stellate   ( ) Galeazzi
( ) torus   ( ) fatigue   ( ) Monteggia
( ) dislocated   ( ) epiphyseal   ( ) pathologic
( ) avulsion   ( ) Colles   ( ) subluxed
( ) boxer   ( ) stress   ( ) Smith
( ) Bennett   ( ) Pott

22. (   )   List six radiographically important types of arthritis.

23. (   )   Describe gout, osteoarthritis, and rheumatoid arthritis.

24. (   )   Explain bursitis.

25. (   )   Define spondylolisthesis.

EXERCISE III-1

Complete the blanks in the following statements.

1. Name the type of fracture that occurs at sites of maximum

   stress but without trauma. _fatigue_____

2. What type of arthritis has tophi associated with

   it? _gout_____

3. Where is yellow bone marrow found in the long bones?

   _marrow_____   _cavity_____

4. Name the five functions of the skeleton.

movement   _storage_

protection   _production of red blood_
                    cells

support

5. What is the condition when a vertebra takes on the appearance of the one

above or below it? _transitional_

6. What type of fracture may accompany a dislocated shoulder?

avulsion

7. The main portion, or shaft, of a long bone is called the

diaphysis .

8. Name the six types of synovial joints.

gliding   _saddle_

hinge   _pivot_

condylar   _ball & socket_

9. What type of cell is associated with absorption and removal of

bone? _osteoclast_

10. Name the two divisions of the skeleton.

appendicular   _axial_

11. During arthrography, (positive, negative) ___positive___ contrast media can obscure pathology.

12. Radiography is not as sensitive to bone destruction as ___nuclear___ ___medicine___ because at least ___50___ percent of the bone is destroyed before radiography shows visible changes.

13. Giant cell tumors are also known as ___Osteoclastomas___.

14. As the bone marrow in the spinal column hypertrophies, it exerts pressure on the spinal cord, increasing the possibility of ___paraplegia___. This occurs in which primary malignant tumor? ___multiple___ ___mylomea___

15. What type of fracture causes the cortex to fold back onto itself? ___torus___

EXERCISE III-2

Mark the following statements "T" for true or "F" for false. If it is a false statement, reword it to make it true by changing the incorrect portions.

___F___ 1. Production of red blood cells occurs in ~~yellow~~ red bone marrow.

___T___ 2. A "fat pad" sign is indicative of a fractured elbow.

___T___ 3. CT can reveal lesions, fractures, bone mineralization, and soft tissue involvement.

___F___ 4. ~~Cortical~~ spongy bone stores ~~red~~ yellow bone marrow.

_T_ 5. Increased uric acid in the blood causes tophi, which is characteristic of gout.

_F_ 6. Osteoblasts are ~~the bone reabsorber cells of the body.~~ form bone matrix

_T_ 7. A Smith fracture is of the distal radius with forward displacement.

_T_ 8. In fibrous dysplasia, the radiograph shows a well-circumscribed lesion with thin bands of sclerosis.

_F_ 9. ~~Nuclear medicine~~ arthograms studies can demonstrate the joint space, menisci, ligaments, and cartilage.

_T_ 10. Sacralization occurs when L-5 fuses with the sacrum.

_T_ 11. Ossification is the process of bone replacing hyaline cartilage.

_F_ 12. Brown tumors are associated with ~~rickets.~~ renal osteodistrophes

_F_ 13. Areas of dead bone are termed callus.

_F_ 14. Primary bone malignancies are the most common type of tumor found. metastatic

_T_ 15. Bursitis is caused by excess stress on the joint.

EXERCISE III-3

Circle the letter in front of the correct answer.

1. What condition has a nidus surrounded by dense bone?
   A. osteochondroma
   B. osteoid osteoma
   C. osteosis
   D. osteomalacia

2. Neoplastic bone changes involve
   A. benign tumors
   B. diffuse disease
   C. malignant tumors
   D. a combination of the above

3. An abnormal decrease in bone density resulting from failure of the osteoblasts to produce bone is called
   A. osteoporosis
   B. osteomyelitis
   C. osteochondritis
   D. osteopetrosis

4. A fracture that involves the pulling loose of bone by a ligament or tendon is called
   A. oblique
   B. fatigue
   C. Colles
   D. avulsion

5. If the bone fragment pierces the overlying skin, the fracture is said to be
   A. comminuted
   B. compound
   C. pathologic
   D. compressed

6. The substance that grows between the ends of bone fragments and is eventually changed into osseous tissue in the healing process is known as
   A. callus
   B. cicatrix
   C. collagen
   D. sequestrum

7. A transverse fracture of the distal radius with posterior displacement of the fragment is called
   A. Pott
   B. boxer
   C. greenstick
   D. Colles

8. A fracture that results from disease is known as
   A. pathologic
   B. crepitus
   C. trauma
   D. blowout

9. Arthritis characterized by inflammation and thickening of the synovial membrane, swelling, joint dysfunction, and bilateral joint involvement is known as
   A. osteoarthritis
   B. rheumatoid arthritis
   C. gout
   D. Reiter syndrome

10. A malignant neoplastic disease occurring in young children is
   A. osteogenic sarcoma
   B. Ewing sarcoma
   C. multiple myeloma
   D. chondrosarcoma

11. What type of fracture occurs when one fragment end is driven up into the other fragment end as in a telescope?
   A. compression
   B. impacted
   C. compound
   D. avulsion

12. Aging and postmenopausal hormonal changes are the major cause of
   A. osteoporosis
   B. osteogenesis imperfecta
   C. osteopetrosis
   D. osteomalacia

13. This fracture involves the medial and lateral malleoli of the ankle with dislocation of the joint.
   A. stress
   B. Colles
   C. Pott
   D. avulsion

14. Which disease is associated with a brown tumor?
   A. renal osteodystrophy
   B. achondroplasia
   C. rickets
   D. Brodie abscess

15. Which of the following lines the marrow cavity?
   A. periosteum
   B. endosteum
   C. bone marrow
   D. diaphysis

16. Which are manifestations of achondroplasia?
   (1) dwarfism   (2) bulky forehead   (3) lordosis
   A. 1 and 2
   B. 1 and 3
   C. 2 and 3
   D. 1, 2, and 3

17. Which procedure is done under sterile technique?
   A. CT
   B. MRI
   C. arthrogram
   D. nuclear medicine

18. Compression fractures of the thoracic spine and fractures of the hip are common in women with
   A. osteomalacia
   B. osteopetrosis
   C. osteoporosis
   D. osteosarcoma

19. Which are types of chondromas?
   (1) exostosis   (2) enchondroma   (3) chondrosarcoma
   A. 1 and 2
   B. 1 and 3
   C. 2 and 3
   D. 1, 2, and 3

20. Which fracture does *not* belong?
    A. Colles
    B. Smith
    C. Monteggia
    D. Pott

21. Complications such as conjunctivitis and ulcerations on the hand and feet are associated with
    A. rheumatoid arthritis
    B. tuberculous arthritis
    C. Reiter syndrome
    D. ankylosing spondylitis

22. The term used when fractures are placed in as close to normal position as possible is
    A. fixation
    B. splinting
    C. traction
    D. reduction

23. Which statement is *incorrect?*
    A. rickets is a metabolic bone disease
    B. osteopetrosis is a marble bone disease
    C. impaction relates to a bone that is splintered
    D. skull sutures are synarthrodial joints

24. When the "fat pad sign" is seen on a lateral radiograph of a traumatized elbow,
    A. fracture should be suspected
    B. joint dislocation should be suspected
    C. nothing is wrong as this is normal on lateral radiographs
    D. infection has set in

25. Inflammation of the vertebrae would be referred to as
    A. spondylolisthesis
    B. spondylitis
    C. spondylalgia
    D. spondylolysis

26. A stellate fracture may involve the
    (1) patella   (2) sternum   (3) skull
    A. 1 and 2 only
    B. 1 and 3 only
    C. 2 and 3 only
    D. 1, 2, and 3

27. A tumor composed of both cartilaginous and bony substance is an
    A. osteosarcoma
    B. osteoblastoma
    C. osteocystoma
    D. osteochondroma

28. Which of the following are classified as irregular bones?
    (1) sphenoid   (2) patellae   (3) lumbar vertebrae
    A.   1 and 2 only
    B.   1 and 3 only
    C.   2 and 3 only
    D.   1, 2, and 3

29. All of the following are part of the axial skeleton of the body *except* the
    A.   skull
    B.   pelvic girdle
    C.   thoracic cage
    D.   vertebral column

30. Which of the following shows blurred bilateral SI joints and a "bamboo" spine?
    A.   rheumatoid spondylitis
    B.   rheumatoid arthritis
    C.   osteoarthritis
    D.   hypertrophic arthritis

EXERCISE III-4

Match each of the following with the correct definition by placing the letter of the answer in the space provided. Each question has only one correct answer.

A. osteopetrosis

B. bursitis

C. osteoporosis

D. osteomyelitis

E. Ewing sarcoma

F. osteitis deformans

G. multiple myeloma

H. achondroplasia

I. osteoarthritis

J. osteosarcoma

K. rheumatoid arthritis

L. osteochondroma

M. osteogenesis imperfecta

N. osteomalacia

O. osteoclastoma

P. Legg-Calvé-Perthes

Q. avulsion

R. compound

S. compression

T. comminuted

U. Bennett

V. epiphyseal

W. boxer

X. renal osteodystrophy

Y. rheumatoid spondylitis

Z. subluxation

Bennett

1. _U_ fracture of the base of first metacarpal

Legg Clave

2. _P_ flattened femoral head is associated with this

Renal Ostedystroph

3. _X_ salt and pepper skull

Ostegenieneas perfata

4. _M_ brittle bone disease

Osteo malacia

5. _N_ caused by vitamin deficiency

Osteopetrosis

6. _A_ marble bone disease

Subluxation

7. _Z_ partial dislocation

Osteomylitis

8. _D_ infection of the bone and its marrow

Compression

9. _S_ fracture of one bone where the two ends are pressed toward the middle

10. __I__ most common type of arthritis   *osteoarthritis*

11. __G__ most common primary malignant bone tumor   *multiple myloma*

12. __N__ abnormal decrease in bone density owing to lack of calcium   *osteomalacia*

13. __H__ failure of cartilage to form properly, which leads to dwarfism
achondroplasia

14. __C__ associated with kidney stones owing to excretion of calcium in the urine
osteoperosis

15. __F__ also called Paget disease   *osteitis deformans*

16. __L__ benign tumor arising from the cortex of the bone and capped by cartilage   *osteochondroma*

17. __E__ may be misdiagnosed as osteomyelitis
Ewing sarcoma

18. __E__ classic appearance of "onion peel"   *Ewing Sarcoma*

19. __O__ classic appearance of "soap bubbles"   *osteoclastoma*

20. __X__ classic appearance of "rugger jersey" spine   *Renal osteodystrophy*

21. __F__ classic appearance of "cotton wool" skull
osteitis deformans

22. __G__ classic appearance of "swiss cheese" skull
multiple myloma

23. __J__ classic appearance of "sunray"
osteosarcoma

24. __I__ classic appearance of "spurring" at joint space
osteoarthritis

25. __B__ most common nonarthritic joint ailment
bursitis

26. __K__ leads to boutonniere or swan neck deformity
rheumatoid arthritis

27. __T__ fracture with multiple fragments
comminuted

28. __W__ fracture of the fifth metacarpal
boxer

29. __Q__ "chip" fracture that can occur with dislocations   *avulsion*

30 __K__

CHAPTER III SELF-TEST

There are 50 possible points on this self-test. Score it against the answers found in the exercises. A score of 47 points or higher indicates mastery and retention of this material.

Complete the blanks in the following statements.

1. Where will yellow bone marrow be found in the long bones?

   marrow cavity

2. Name the six types of synovial joints.

   gliding   *hinge*

   saddle   *pivot*

   ball & socket   *condylar*

3. What type of fracture causes the cortex to fold back onto itself?

   Torus

4. During arthrography, _____ *positive* _____ contrast media can obscure pathology.

5. Name the five functions of the skeleton.

   positive storage   *support*

   protecture   *production of Red Blood c.*

   movement

6. What type of fracture may accompany a dislocated shoulder?

avulsion

7. Radiography is not as sensitive to bone destruction as

nuclear   _medicine_ because at

least _____ 50 _____ percent of the bone is
destroyed before radiography shows visible changes.

8. Name the two divisions of the skeleton.

axial and

appendicular

9. What is the condition when a vertebra takes on the appearance of the one

above or below it? _transitional_

10. What type of cell is associated with absorption and removal of bone?

Osteoclast

11. Name the type of fracture that occurs at sites of maximum stress but without

trauma. _fatigue_

12. As the bone marrow in the spinal column hypertrophies, it exerts pressure on
the spinal cord, increasing the possibility

of _paraplegia_ . This occurs in which primary

malignant tumor? _multiple myeloma_

Mark the following statements "T" for true or "F" for false.

_T_ 13. In fibrous dysplasia, the radiograph shows a well-circumscribed lesion with thin bands of sclerosis.

_F_ 14. Production of red blood cells occurs in ~~yellow~~ *red* bone marrow.

_F_ 15. Brown tumors are associated with ~~rickets.~~ *renal osteodystrophy*

_F_ 16. ~~Nuclear medicine~~ *arthrography* studies can demonstrate the joint space, menisci, ligaments, and cartilage.

_F_ 17. Osteo~~b~~*c*lasts are the bone reabsorber cells of the body.

_T_ 18. A "fat pad" sign is indicative of a fractured elbow.

_F_ 19. Areas of dead bone are termed ~~callus~~.

_T_ 20. Bursitis is caused by excess stress on the joint.

_T_ 21. Ossification is the process of bone replacing hyaline cartilage.

_T_ 22. Increased uric acid in the blood causes tophi, which are characteristic of gout.

_T_ 23. A Smith fracture is of the distal radius with forward displacement.

_F_ 24. Primary bone malignancies are the most common type of tumor found. *metatic*

Circle the letter in front of the correct answer.

25. A fracture that involves the pulling loose of bone by a ligament or tendon is called
    A. oblique
    B. fatigue
    C. Colles
    D. avulsion

26. What type of fracture occurs when one fragment end is driven up into the other end, as in a telescope?
    A. compression
    B. impacted
    C. compound
    D. avulsion

27. Which fracture involves the medial and lateral malleoli of the ankle with dislocation of the joint?
    A. stress
    B. Colles
    C. Pott
    D. avulsion

28. If the bone fragment pierces the overlying skin, the fracture is said to be
    A. comminuted
    B. compound
    C. pathologic
    D. compressed

29. A transverse fracture of the distal radius with posterior displacement of the fragment is called
    A. Pott
    B. boxer
    C. greenstick
    D. Colles

30. Compression fractures of the thoracic spine and fractures of the hip are common in women with
    A. osteomalacia
    B. osteopetrosis
    C. osteoporosis
    D. osteosarcoma

31. Which fracture does *not* belong?
    A. Colles
    B. Smith
    C. Monteggia
    D. Pott

32. An abnormal decrease in bone density resulting from failure of the osteoblasts to produce bone is called
    A. osteoporosis
    B. osteomyelitis
    C. osteochondritis
    D. osteopetrosis

33. A fracture that results from disease is known as
    A. pathologic
    B. crepitus
    C. trauma
    D. blowout

34. Which are manifestations of achondroplasia?
    (1) dwarfism   (2) bulky forehead   (3) lordosis
    A. 1 and 2
    B. 1 and 3
    C. 2 and 3
    D. 1, 2, and 3

35. Neoplastic bone changes involve
    A. benign tumors
    B. diffuse disease
    C. malignant tumors
    D. a combination of the above

36. Which of the following shows blurred bilateral SI joints and a "bamboo" spine?
    A. rheumatoid spondylitis
    B. rheumatoid arthritis
    C. osteoarthritis
    D. hypertrophic arthritis

37. Arthritis characterized by inflammation and thickening of the synovial membranes, swelling, joint dysfunction, and bilateral joint involvement is known as
    A. osteoarthritis
    B. rheumatoid arthritis
    C. gout
    D. Reiter syndrome

Match each of the following with the correct definition by placing the letter of the answer in the space provided. Each question has only one correct answer.

A. osteopetrosis

B. renal osteodystrophy

C. osteoporosis

D. rheumatoid spondylitis

E. Ewing sarcoma

F. osteitis deformans

G. multiple myeloma

H. osteosarcoma

I. subluxation

J. osteoclastoma

K. Legg-Calvé-Perthes

L. osteogenesis/imperfecta

M. rheumatoid arthritis

N. compression

O. comminuted

P. Bennett

38. _E_ classic appearance of "onion peel" *Ewing sarcoma*

39. _L_ brittle bone disease *osteogenesis/ imperfecta*

40. _M_ also called Paget disease *rheumatoid arthritis*

41. _H_ classic appearance of "sunray" *osteosarcoma*

42. _K_ flattened femoral head is associated with this *Legg Clave Perthes*

43. _J_ classic appearance of "soap bubbles" *Osteoclastoma*

44. _B_ salt and pepper skull *renal osteo dystrophy*

45. _F_ classic appearance of "cotton wool" skull *cotton (osteitis deformans*

46. _I_ partial dislocation *subluxation*

47. _B_ classic appearance of "rugger jersey" spine *renal osteodystropy*

48. _A_ marble bone disease *osteopetrosis*

49. _M_ leads to boutonniere or swan neck deformity *rheumatoid arthritis*

50. _P_ fracture of the base of first metacarpal *Bennett*

CHAPTER IV

Hepatobiliary System

Rationale

Diseases of the biliary system affect many Americans every year. Demonstration of such diseases is often difficult and, in some cases, occurs as an incidental finding on an unrelated examination. The technologist who has met the challenge of mastering the difficult biliary ductal anatomy is a boon to the radiologist. These technologists can be "free thinkers" and provide the physician with the radiograph that has just enough obliquity to demonstrate that small piece of calcium away from bowel gas.

The many special radiographic procedures that are used to demonstrate the biliary ductal system must be completely understood by the technologist if he or she is to be of assistance to the physician. Understanding every aspect of these procedures eliminates any guess work. The radiographer must know when pathologic conditions require a change in technique or when a procedure requires modification to facilitate the examination and aid in patient comfort.

Objectives

1. ( ) Identify the right, left, caudate, and quadrate lobes of the liver.

2. ( ) Determine the falciform ligament and ligament of teres on a drawing.

3. ( ) Describe Riedel lobe.

4. ( ) List the three portions of the gallbladder.

5. ( ) Explain the significance of Hartmann pouch.

6. ( ) Explain the purpose of the spiral valve of Heister.

7. ( ) Draw and label the biliary ducts and the pancreatic ducts.

8. ( ) Identify from a drawing the four areas of the pancreas.

9. ( ) List at least five functions of the liver.

10. ( ) Name the four liver function tests described in the text.

11. ( ) Explain how the gallbladder concentrates bile.

12. ( ) Describe the two separate functions of the pancreas.

13. ( ) Name the hormones and enzymes produced by the pancreas.

14. ( ) Explain the impact of the function of the liver on the body.

15. ( ) List the three special imaging modalities used to demonstrate the liver.

16. (　) Name two nuclear medicine studies on the gallbladder.

17. (　) Explain why ultrasound is not the best study for the pancreas.

18. Describe each of the following:

    (　) IVC   (　) ERCP
    (　) T-tube   (　) fatty meal
    (　) PTC   (　) operative cholangiography
    (　) OCG

19. (　) Define cirrhosis.

20. (　) Describe the impact cirrhosis has on the function of the liver.

21. (　) Name all types of viral hepatitis.

22. (　) Describe toxic and deficiency hepatitis.

23. (　) List the two types of medical jaundice.

24. (　) Explain the difference between obstructive and nonobstructive jaundice.

25. (　) Identify three types of congenital anomalies of the gallbladder.

26. (　) List and describe the types of gallstones.

27. (　) Name two complications of gallstones.

28. (　) Describe the differences between acute and chronic cholecystitis.

29. (　) Define enzymatic necrosis.

30. (　) List and describe the two types of pancreatitis.

31. (　) Identify neoplasms of the liver and pancreas.

32. (　) Describe the impact that pancreatitis has on the function of the pancreas.

EXERCISE IV-1

Complete the blanks in the following statements.

1. Name the condition that sets pancreatic inflammation apart from other organ

inflammation. *enzymatic necrosis*

2. Which special imaging modality can detect cancer of the pancreas with almost

100% accuracy? _____CT_____

3. What is the medical term for

gallstones? _____Cholilithiasis_____

4. What is the medical term for inflammation of the

gallbladder? _____Cholecystitis_____

5. What is the medical term for inflammation of the bile

ducts? _____Cholangitis_____

6. What type of jaundice is characterized by the presence of a

gallstone? _____Obstructive (Surgical)_____

7. Ninety percent of all gallstones are caused by too

much _____Cholesterol_____ .

8. How long does it take from the ingestion of a cholecystagogue until the

gallbladder contracts and empties? _____≈ 30 minutes_____

9. What enzyme from the bowel initiates gallbladder

contraction? _____Cholecystikinin_____

10. What causes density of gallstones? _____Calcium_____

11. Name four laboratory function tests for the liver in a jaundiced patient.

SGOT   alkaline phosphatase

SGPT   serum bilirubin

12. What is the major cause of cirrhosis? alcoholism

leonix

13. Removal of the gallbladder by surgery is

termed cholecystectomy.

14. List three procedures that can visualize the biliary ductal system.

CT   PTC

ultrasound

15. Which inflammatory process of the liver is caused by fecal

us   contamination? hepatitis A

A - D

A - G

16. Chronic cholecystitis may cause the gallbladder wall to calcify. This condition

is known as porcelin gallbladder.

17. Enzymatic necrosis is associated with which pathologic

process? pancreatitis

18. Which imaging modality is now used almost exclusively to visualize the

gallbladder and its biliary ducts? ultrasound

19. Name two pathologic reasons that would cause nonvisualization of the gallbladder.

   blockage of cystic ducts   blockage of hepatic duct

20. List the three types of cells found in the pancreas from which tumors might arise.

   acinar cells   island of Langerhand
   beta cells

21. What is the major component of bile? *Water*

22. Why is the T-tube clamped one day before the scheduled T-tube examination? *to concentrate the bile in the tube to prevent air accumulation*

23. What is the most common cause of nonvisualization of the gallbladder in OCG? *poor patient preparation*

24. Identify the anatomic parts indicated.

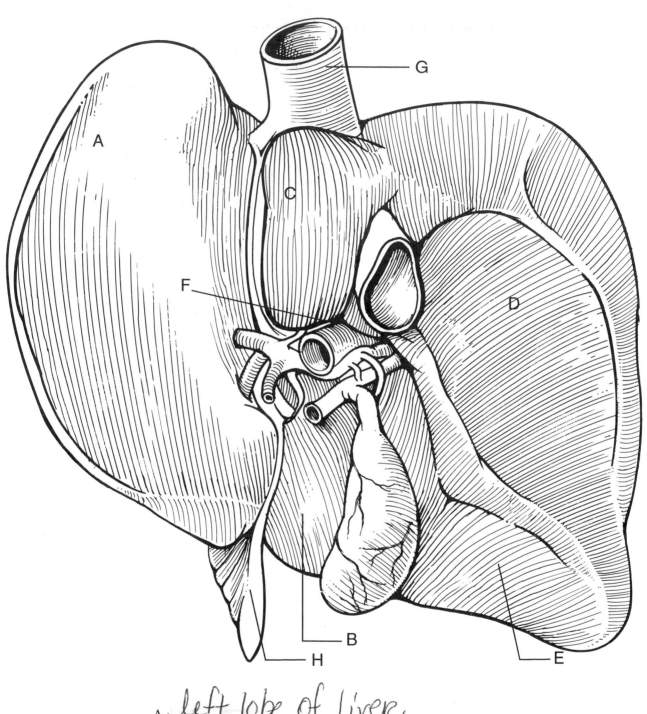

A. *left lobe of liver*

B. *quadrate lobe,*

C. *caudate lobe,*

D. *Right lobe of liver*

E. *Reidals lobe of liver*

F. _~~portal vein~~_

G. _~~IVC~~_

H. _~~falciform ligament~~_

EXERCISE IV-2

Mark the following statements "T" for true or "F" for false. If it is a false statement, reword it to make it true by changing the incorrect portions.

___T___ 1. Neo-Cholex is given to determine if the gallbladder is functioning.

___F___ 2. Nutrients go to the liver ~~from the small bowel~~ by way of the ~~inferior vena cava~~ *portal* *vein*

___F___ *PTC* 3. ~~IVC~~ involves a needle inserted directly into the biliary tree, withdrawing bile, and injecting contrast material.

___F___ 4. The biliary system includes the gallbladder, *liver* ~~pancreas~~, and ~~spleen~~. *bile ducts*

___T___ 5. The Kupffer cells of the liver destroy worn out red blood cells.

___F___ 6. A fatty liver may be caused by ~~obesity~~. *cirrhosis*

___T___ 7. The most common type of gallstone is the radiolucent type.

___F___ 8. Cholegrafin is used for a ~~T-tube examination~~. *IVC* ∟ *Renografin, Conray Isovue*

___T___ 9. A skinny needle is used in PTC.

___F___ 10. A nonfunctioning gallbladder can be determined by ~~ultrasonography~~. *Nuclear Medicine*

___F___ 11. The spiral valve of Heister is located in the common ~~hepatic~~ duct. *cystic*

___T___ 12. Gallstones can lodge in the cystic duct.

___T___ 13. Cholecystokinin causes the gallbladder to empty.

___T___ 14. Bile-evac is used in a fatty meal study of the gallbladder.

___F___ 15. The ~~gallbladder~~ produces bile. *liver*

_F_ 16. A PIPIDA scan is a nuclear medicine study of the ~~pancreas~~.

gall bladder & ducts

_F_ 17. Detoxification of substances takes place in the ~~pancreas~~. liver

_T_ 18. ERCP is contraindicated in acute pancreatitis.

_f_ 19. Hepatomas are best demonstrated by ~~ultrasonography~~. CT & angiography

_f_ 20. ~~Adenomas~~ are the most common neoplasm of the pancreas. adenocarcinoma

_T_ 21. Pancreatic pseudocysts can be found anywhere in the body.

_T_ 22. The gallbladder will probably not visualize on OCG if the bilirubin is higher than 4 mg/100 mL of serum.

_T_ 23. The liver controls the level of glucose in the blood.

_T_ 24. Barium studies can show pathology of the pancreas.

_f_ 25. The patient must remain NPO for approximately ~~8~~ 10 hours following ERCP.

EXERCISE IV-3

Circle the letter in front of the correct answer.

1. Which examination is done by inserting a needle into the biliary ducts?
   A. PAP
   B. PTC
   C. ERCP
   D. ESWL

2. Which examination has been replaced by modern technology and is no longer performed?
   A. ESWL
   B. PTC
   C. IVC
   D. ERCP

3. Radiolucent gallstones are composed of
   A. cholesterol
   B. calcium
   C. mineral salts
   D. bilirubin

4. Which of the following is secreted by the pancreas?
   A. pepsin
   B. gastrin
   C. trypsin
   D. cholecystokinin

5. Which of the following procedures assesses all functions of the gallbladder?
   A. cholecystography paired with a double dose
   B. cholecystography paired with a fatty meal examination
   C. ERCP and CT
   D. IVC paired with an ultrasound examination

6. Which of the following procedures carries the lowest risk to the patient?
   A. PTC
   B. ERCP
   C. operative cholangiogram
   D. OCG

7. Stratification of gallstones can be visualized radiographically by obtaining which of the following positions?
   A. anterior oblique
   B. posterior oblique
   C. erect and decubitus
   D. lateral

8. The portal vein is formed by the union of the
   A. splenic and superior mesenteric veins
   B. hepatic and inferior mesenteric veins
   C. splenic and gastric veins
   D. superior mesenteric and cystic veins

9. Which of the following is a cholecystagogue?
   A. Renografin
   B. Cholex
   C. Conray
   D. Hypaque

10. Which of the following areas would *not* be demonstrated on an IVC?
    A. common bile duct
    B. duct of Santorini
    C. hepatic duct
    D. cystic duct

11. If hemoglobin cannot be excreted in bile and eliminated in feces, the result is
    A. anemia
    B. leukemia
    C. jaundice
    D. a bleeding tendency

12. Blockage of the cystic duct causes the gallbladder to increase in size, causing a condition known as
    A. paralysis
    B. cholecystitis
    C. cholelithiasis
    D. hydrops

13. The portion of the pancreas that extends toward the spleen is the
    A. head
    B. neck
    C. body
    D. tail

14. Which of the following is the most dependent portion of the gallbladder?
    A. Hartmann pouch
    B. fundus
    C. body
    D. cystic duct

15. The common bile duct drains into the
    A. cystic duct
    B. hepatic duct
    C. stomach
    D. ampulla of Vater

16. Which of the following statements is *false*?
    A. cirrhosis may be due to a viral hepatitis
    B. complications of cirrhosis are ascites and esophageal varices
    C. cirrhosis is not common in the United States
    D. CT films of a liver with cirrhosis show lesions

17. Which of the following is a rare form of hepatitis in the United States?
    A. hepatitis A
    B. hepatitis C
    C. hepatitis D
    D. hepatitis E

18. Which of the following congenital anomalies of the gallbladder consists of an internal septum dividing it into two chambers?
    A. duplication of the gallbladder
    B. bilobed gallbladder
    C. hourglass gallbladder
    D. Phrygian cap gallbladder

19. Metastatic carcinomas of the liver occur from primary sources of all of the following *except*
    A. lung
    B. gastrointestinal tract
    C. breast
    D. endometrium

20. Which carcinoma ranks high among fatalities in the United States?
    A. primary hepatic carcinoma
    B. carcinoma of the pancreas
    C. carcinoma of the gallbladder
    D. cholangiocarcinoma

EXERCISE IV-4

Match each of the following with the correct definition by placing the letter of the answer in the space provided. Each question has only one correct answer.

A. cirrhosis

B. phrygian cap

C. jaundice

D. acute pancreatitis

E. cholangiocarcinoma

F. carcinoma

G. hepatitis

H. hepatomas

I. chronic pancreatitis

J. cholangitis

1. __F__ 75% of all cases occur in the head of the pancreas   *Carcinoma*

2. __D__ a pseudocyst may be associated with this condition   *acute pancreatitis*

3. __I__ this disease eventually causes calcification to occur in the pancreas
chronic pancreatitis

4. __A__ most common cause of this condition is alcohol-abuse
cirrhosis

5. __B__ fundus of the gallbladder folded over onto the body
phrygian cap

6. __G__ inflammation of the liver cells
hepatitis

7. __C__ the result of bilirubin in the blood
jaundice

8. __A__ the end stage of liver disease
cirrhosis

Match the anatomic part with the correct name.

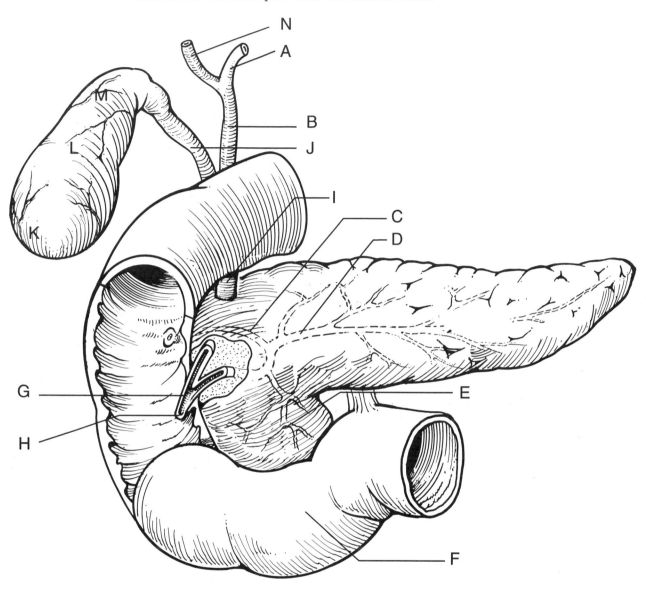

9. __I__ common bile duct

10. __M__ neck of gallbladder

11. __B__ common hepatic duct

12. __K__ fundus of gallbladder

13. __H__ sphincter of Oddi

14. __D__ duct of Wirsung

15. __G__ ampulla of Vater

16. __J__ cystic duct

17. __N__ right hepatic duct

18. __F__ duodenum

19. __L__ body of gallbladder

20. __A__ left hepatic duct

CHAPTER IV SELF-TEST

There are 50 possible points on this self-test. Score it against the answers found in the exercises. A score of 47 points or higher indicates mastery and retention of this material.

Complete the blanks in the following statements.

1. Ninety percent of all gallstones are caused by too much ___cholesteral___ .

90% of all gallstones are caused by too much cholesterol

2. Which special imaging modality can detect cancer of the pancreas with almost

   100% accuracy? _CT_

3. Chronic cholecystitis may cause the gallbladder wall to calcify. This condition

   is known as _porcelin gallbladder_

   porcelin gallbladder

4. Name four laboratory function tests for the liver in a jaundiced patient.

   _____   _____

   _____   _____

5. What is the most common cause of nonvisualization of the gallbladder in oral

   cholecystography? _poor patient prep_

6. Name the condition that sets pancreatic inflammation apart from other organ

   inflammation. _enzymatic necrosis_

7. What is the medical term for inflammation of the

   gallbladder? _cholecystitis_

   cholecystitis

8. What is the major component of bile? _H2O_

   water

9. List three procedures that can visualize the biliary ductal system.

   _CT_   _ultrasound_

   Nuclear Medicine

10. What type of jaundice is characterized by the presence of a

    gallstone? _Obstructive (surgical)_

11. How long does it take from the ingestion of a cholecystagogue until the

    gallbladder contracts and empties? _30 min / 30 minutes_

12. What is the major cause of cirrhosis? _alcoholism_
    alcoholism

13. What causes density of gallstones? _calcium / calcium_

14. What is the medical term for gallstones?

    Cholelithiasis   _cholelithiasis_

15. What enzyme from the bowel initiates gallbladder

    contraction? _CCK_   _CCK_

Mark the following statements "T" for true or "F" for false.

_T_ 16. Gallstones can lodge in the cystic duct.

_F_ 17. *PTC* ~~IVC~~ involves a needle inserted directly into the biliary tree, withdrawing
       bile, and injecting contrast material.

_F_ 18. ~~Cholegrafin~~ is used for a ~~T-tube examination~~. *IVC*
       Cholegraffin is used for a IVC

_T_ 19. The liver controls the level of glucose in the blood.

_F_ 20. Detoxification of substances takes place in the ~~pancreas~~. *liver*

_F_ 21. The patient must remain NPO for approximately ~~8~~ *10* hours following ERCP.

_F_ 22. Fatty liver may be caused by ~~obesity~~. *@ cirrhosis*

_F_ 23. The spiral valve of Heister is located in the common ~~hepatic~~ duct. *cystic*

___F___ 24. A PIPIDA scan is a nuclear medicine study of the ~~pancreas~~. *gallbladder & ducts*

___T___ 25. Neo-Cholex is given to determine if the gallbladder is functioning.

___F___ 26. ~~Adenomas~~ *adenocarcinomas* are the most common neoplasm of the pancreas.

___T___ 27. A nonfunctioning gallbladder can be determined by ultrasonography.

___T___ 28. The most common type of gallstone is the radiolucent type.

___T___ 29. The gallbladder will probably not visualize on OCG if the bilirubin is higher than 4 mg/100 mL of serum.

___F___ 30. The ~~gallbladder~~ *liver* produces bile.

Circle the letter in front of the correct answer.

31. Which of the following is secreted by the pancreas?
    A. pepsin
    B. gastrin
    C. trypsin
    D. cholecystokinin

32. The portion of the pancreas that extends toward the spleen is the
    A. head
    B. neck
    C. body
    D. tail

33. Stratification of gallstones can be visualized radiographically by obtaining which of the following positions?
    A. anterior oblique
    B. posterior oblique
    C. erect and decubitus
    D. lateral

34. Which carcinoma ranks high among fatalities in the United States?
    A. primary hepatic carcinoma
    B. carcinoma of the pancreas
    C. carcinoma of the gallbladder
    D. cholangiocarcinoma

35. Which examination is done by inserting a needle into the biliary ducts?
    A. PAP
    B. PTC
    C. ERCP
    D. ESWL

36. If hemoglobin cannot be excreted in bile and eliminated in the feces, the result is
    A. anemia
    B. leukemia
    C. jaundice
    D. a bleeding tendency

37. Metastatic carcinomas of the liver arise from primary sites of all of the following *except*
    A. lung
    B. gastrointestinal tract
    C. breast
    D. endometrium

38. Which examination has been replaced by modern technology and is no longer performed?
    A. ESWL
    B. PTC
    C. IVC
    D. ERCP

39. Which of the following procedures carries the lowest risk to the patient?
    A. PTC
    B. ERCP
    C. operative cholangiogram
    D. OCG

40. The common bile duct drains into the
    A. cystic duct
    B. hepatic duct
    C. stomach
    D. ampulla of Vater

Match the anatomic part with the correct name.

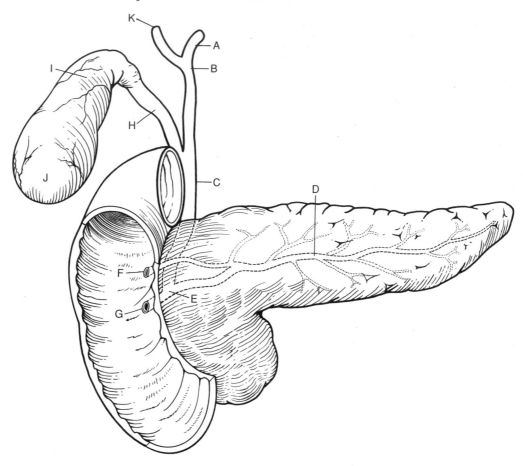

41. __C__ common bile duct

42. __A__ left hepatic duct

43. __D__ duct of Wirsung

44. __H__ cystic duct

45. __K__ right hepatic duct

46. __I__ neck of gallbladder

47. __E__ ampulla of Vater

48. __G__ sphinter of Oddi

49. __F__ duct of Santorini

50. __B__ common hepatic duct

Gastrointestinal System

Rationale

The role of the radiographer in fluoroscopy has changed from that of assistant to performer. In 1994, at its annual conference, the American Society of Radiologic Technologists (ASRT) adopted resolutions that incorporated fluoroscopy of the gallbladder and terminal ileum and arthrography of the knee and shoulder to be within the scope of practice for a radiographer. As such, radiographers must be prepared to be more responsible as they take on a more critical role. As technology has changed, radiographers have taken on the responsibility of performing many fluoroscopic examinations either in the presence of a radiologist or under the physician's direction.

In areas (e.g., different exams other than those listed, geographic locations) where the radiologist is still the fluoroscopist, it is the role of the radiographer to assist the radiologist during fluoroscopy. The radiographer must be able to anticipate the physician's needs during a radiographic examination and be ready to accommodate them. In addition, the patient must be attended to. Professionalism is required at all times to provide for the patient's comfort and maintain his or her dignity.

No matter what role the radiographer has (fluoroscopist or assistant), it is his or her responsibility to understand the various pathologic conditions and the patient's physiologic response to these conditions. Should contrast material be warmed? What type of catheters are necessary? Will the patient experience electrolyte imbalance or perhaps further dehydration? The patient's well-being during the examination and possibly the patient's diagnosis depend on the skill of the radiographer.

Objectives

1. (   )   Identify the esophageal hiatus and cardiac orifice.

2. (   )   Determine the fundus, body, curvatures, angular notch, and pylorus of the stomach on a drawing.

3. (   )   List the four portions of the duodenum.

4. (   )   Name the two other portions of the small bowel.

5. (   )   List the three portions of the large bowel.

6. (   )   Identify the ascending, transverse, flexure, descending, and sigmoid portions of the colon on a drawing.

7. (   )   Describe the portions of the bowel created by the taenia coli.

8. (   )   List the three functions of the stomach.

9. (   )   Name the two things the stomach absorbs.

10. (   )   Describe the three functions of the small bowel.

11. (   )   Name the two things the large bowel absorbs.

12. (   )   Describe a hypotonic duodenography.

13. (   )   Explain why interventional radiography would be used for the gastrointestinal system.

14. (   )   List two congenital anomalies of the esophagus.

15. (   )   Describe how achalasia occurs.

16. (   )   List two types of hiatal hernias.

17. (   )   Explain the significance of Schatzki ring.

18. (   )   Describe the appearance of an intrathoracic stomach.

19. (   )   List the two types of esophageal diverticula and describe the radiographic appearance of each.

20. (   )   Define Barrett esophagus.

21. (   )   Name the classic appearance of esophageal varices.

22. (   )   Explain the cause of the appearance of varices of the esophagus.

23. (   )   Describe the congenital anomaly of pyloric stenosis.

24. (   )   Explain how both types of bezoars occur.

25. (   )   Name the two types of peptic ulcers.

26. (   )   Describe the three types of malignant tumors of the stomach.

27. (   )   Define malabsorption syndrome.

28. (   )   Explain the difference between mechanical and ileus bowel obstructions.

29. (   )   Describe Crohn's disease.

30. Describe the following large bowel pathologies:

    (   )   Hirschsprung disease   (   )   volvulus
    (   )   intussusception   (   )   cathartic colon

31. (   )   Explain the differences between granulomatous and ulcerative colitis.

32. ( ) List two types of polyps of the large bowel.

33. ( ) Describe the appearance of annular lesions of the bowel.

EXERCISE V-1

Complete the blanks in the following statements.

1. Malignant tumors of the esophagus demonstrate a definite division between normal tissue and tumor. This division is termed

Shelving Malignant tumors of the esophagus demonstrate a definite diversion b/t normal tissue and tumor is called shelving.

2. Name the <u>congenital diverticulum</u> that represents the persistence of the <u>yolk</u>

sac. _Meckel Diverticulum_

yolk sac — Meckel Diverticulum

3. What medical term denotes difficulty in swallowing?

dysphagia

difficult swallowing — dysphagia

4. The pathologic condition in which the wall of the <u>gallbladder</u> is <u>calcified</u>

is _porcelin gallbladder_.

gallbladder calcified — porcelin gallbladder

5. In what part of the <u>small bowel</u> will a congenital diverticulum be

found? _ileum_

find a congenital diverticulum in the | ileum |

6. A condition wherein the bowel twists over onto itself is called

volvulus ⇒ volvulus

7. Hemorrhoids are the result of enlargement of which part of the

rectum? _rectal columns_

Rectal columns ⟵ = Hemorrhoids are caused by enlarged.

8. Of the two types of intussusception, which is secondary to some type of mass in the lumen of the bowel? *adult*

9. Name the two categories of esophageal diverticula.

pulsion   *traction*

10. What condition is due to taking too many laxatives for too long a period of time? *cathartic colon*

11. What disease is due to reflux esophagitis, which causes ulcerations? *Barrett esophagus*

12. Name the three parts of the large bowel.

cecum   *rectum*

colon

13. Name the most frequent site of gastric ulcers.

lesser curvature

14. Name two types of bezoars.

phytobezoar   *trichobezoar*

15. The patient must perform what maneuver to demonstrate gastric reflux into the esophagus? *Valsalva*

16. The radiograph shows distended loops of bowel in the central portion of the film in what type of obstruction? *small bowel*

17. The entire large bowel has three bands of muscle fibers running its length. These muscle fibers are called the *tainea coli* .

18. What procedure uses barium and air to study the duodenum? *hypotonic duodenography*

19. What interventional procedure uses balloons to occlude or dilate blood vessels within the gastrointestinal tract? *percutaneous transluminal angicplasty*

20. Why are foreign objects in the esophagus important to identify? *may perforate esophagus and cause an abscess*

21. Duodenal ulcers are more commonly found in which portion of the stomach? *greater curvature*

22. What type of ulcer produces the classic radiographic appearance of a "cloverleaf"? *duodenal*
Cloverleaf — duodenal ulcer

23. Name two congenital anomalies of the large bowel in which there is no opening at the anal canal or no anus.
imperforate anus   rectal atresia

24. Which portion of the digestive tract carries out the processes of digestion and absorption? *small bowel*

25. A passageway between the trachea and the esophagus is known as

a _fistula_____ .

EXERCISE V-2

Mark the following statements "T" for true or "F" for false. If it is a false statement, reword it to make it true by changing the incorrect portions.

T _____ 1. Ulcerative colitis is a diffusely distributed mucosal disease.

T _____ 2. A congenital lack of development of the esophagus at any point is known as atresia.

F _____ 3. Meckel diverticulum is a congenital defect ~~of the esophagus.~~ *found in ileum*

T _____ 4. Any ulcer of the stomach is a peptic ulcer.

F _____ 5. The taenia coli can be seen on the radiograph and demarcates the junction of the two parts of the small bowel. *Ligament of Treitz demarcates the junction*

Ⓣ _____ 6. Hirschsprung disease is caused by the congenital absence of neurons in the colon, which prevents peristalsis.

F _____ 7. Esophageal stricture is due ~~to violent vomiting that overdistends the base of the esophagus.~~ *rupture*

F _____ 8. An example of a traction diverticulum is a ~~Zenker diverticulum.~~ *pulsion tick*

T _____ 9. CT and ultrasonography are useful modalities for demonstrating metastases of abdominal viscera.

F _____ 10. Prolapse occurs when the gastric mucosa is pushed into the ~~ascending colon.~~ *pyloric canal*

F _____ 11. The greatest amount of digestion occurs in the ~~stomach.~~ *small bowel*

FⒻ _____ 12. A 40-year-old patient who has difficulty swallowing is tested for esophageal ~~varices.~~ *esophageal carcina*

T _____ 13. A water siphonage test is used to help determine reflux esophagitis.

T _____ 14. A pharyngeal pouch can become so large as to be outwardly discernible.

F _____ 15. "Shelving" is demonstrated in ~~pyloric stenosis.~~ *esophageal carcinoma*

_T_ 16. The large bowel functions to eliminate waste and absorb water.

_F_ 17. When a portion of the stomach slides above the diaphragm, leaving the gastroesophageal junction in place, the patient is said to have a sliding hernia. _rolling or paraesophageal hernia_

_T_ 18. Esophageal spasms are difficult to diagnose radiographically.

_F_ 19. Pulsion diverticula of the esophagus have a distinctive triangular shape. _traction_

_T_ 20. Pleural effusion can be seen on a patient who has experienced spontaneous rupture of the esophagus.

EXERCISE V-3

Circle the letter in front of the correct answer.

_C_ 1. What radiograph is done to see a displaced stomach owing to retroperitoneal adenopathy?
A. RAO
B. LPO
C. Lateral
D. PA

2. Regional enteritis is also called   _Regional enteritis_
A. Barrett esophagus
B. Cushing disease
C. Crohn's disease   _Chrohn's disease_
D. Zollinger-Ellison disease

_C_ 3. Obstruction of the body of the stomach causes a sign known as the
A. "figure 8"
B. "thumbprint"
C. "hourglass"   _hour glass — Obstruction of stomach_
D. "leather bottle"

4. Which type of adenocarcinoma causes the leather bottle stomach syndrome?
A. papillary
B. ulcerating
C. infiltrating   _leather bottle stomach syndrome — infiltrating_
D. fungating

_A_ 5. What disease shows the "string sign"?
A. regional enteritis
B. Zollinger-Ellison disease
C. esophageal varices
D. paralytic ileus

String sign — Regional enteritis

C 6. The stepladder sign is indicative of
    A. regional enteritis
    B. parasitic small bowel
    C. small bowel obstruction
    D. ulcerative colitis

Stepladder → Small bowel obstruction

7. Portal venous hypertension can result in
    A. hiatal hernia
    B. gastric ulcers
    C. esophageal varices
    D. prolapse of gastric mucosa

8. The condition of one part of the bowel telescoping into another portion is known as
    A. intussusception
    B. volvulus
    C. ileus
    D. obstruction

C 9. Varicose veins of the rectum are termed
    A. polyps
    B. renal columns
    C. hemorrhoids
    D. diverticula

A 10. Annular carcinoma of the colon shows the classic appearance of
    A. apple-core
    B. ground glass
    C. eggshell
    D. bird's beak

apple core – annular carcinoma

B 11. Crohn's disease occurs 80% of the time in which area?
    A. colon
    B. small bowel
    C. stomach
    D. esophagus

small bowel → Chrons disease

A 12. What condition is present when large amounts of air can be seen in dilated loops of small and large bowel?
    A. paralytic ileus
    B. localized ileus
    C. colonic ileus
    D. ischemic ileus

B 13. Outpouchings along the walls of the bowel lumen are termed
    A. ulcers
    B. diverticula
    C. duodenal ulcer
    D. peritoneal ulcer

D 14. The most common site of duodenal ulcers is the
    A. duodenum
    B. pylorus
    C. lesser curvature
    D. greater curvature

C 15. Which is *not* a portion of the duodenum?
    A. ascending portion
    B. superior portion
    C. inferior portion
    D. descending portion

EXERCISE V-4

Match each of the following with the correct definition by placing the letter of the answer in the space provided. Each question has only one correct answer.

A. Crohn's disease

B. achalasia

C. corkscrew esophagus

D. intussusception

E. Hirschsprung disease

F. esophageal varices

G. esophageal web

H. cathartic colon

I. pneumatosis

J. adenocarcinoma of the colon

K. spastic colon

L. pseudotumors

M. pylorospasm

N. hiatal hernia

O. Zollinger-Ellison

P. ulcerative colitis

Q. ischemic colitis

R. sprue

S. gastritis

T. trichobezoar

U. prolapse

1. __R__ shows the moulage sign   Spru   Spru

2. __N__ when the abdominal viscera moves through a defect in the diaphragm
hiatal hernia

3. __O__ most common cause of gastric fold thickening in the fundus of the stomach
Zollinger – Ellison

4. __J__ most commonly occurs in the rectosigmoid area and causes the apple-core sign
adenocarcinoma of the colon

5. __I__ air in the bowel wall
Pneumatosis

6. __A__ inflammatory disease that occurs 80% of the time in the terminal ileum
Chron's deases

7. __K__ due to spasms and shows loss of mucosal markings in the colon
Spastic colon

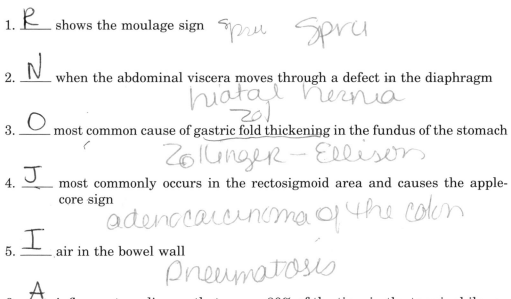

8. _P_ starts in the anus; bowel wall becomes rigid with loss of markings

ulcerative colitis)

9. _C_ tertiary contractions of the esophagus *Corkscrew esophagus*

Cork screw esophagus)

10. _A_ condition that leaves "skipped areas" of normal bowel

Chron's disease)

11. _B_ dilation of the esophagus owing to dysfunction of peristalsis

achlasia achlasia)

12. _R_ also known as celiac disease

sprue Sprue)

13. _P_ has the typical sign of a lead-pipe appearance

ulcerative colitis ulcerative colitis

14. _P_ pseudopolyps are seen with this condition

ulcerative colitis ulcerative colitis

15. _F_ due to increased pressure in the portal venous system and is associated with a large spleen

esophageal varices esophageal varices

16. _U_ due to loose attachments of mucosa, which is pushed through the pyloric channel

prolapse Prolapse)

17. _S_ inflammation of the stomach

gastritis gastritis)

18. _F_ classic appearance of rosary beads

esophageal varices esophageal varices

19. _P_ occurs only 25% of the time in the terminal ileum

ulcerative colitis

20. _P_ colitis that carries a 10% risk of cancer

ulcerative colitis

21. _B_ shows the "rat tail" appearance

achalasia achlasia)

22. _E_ 80% of patients with this disease are males and exhibit failure to thrive and constipation

Hershingpeng dease

23. _T_ foreign body mass such as hair in the stomach

trichobezoar)

24. _R_ disease characterized by poor food absorption and an intolerance of gluten

Sprue)

25. _A_ radiograph demonstrates a cobblestone appearance owing to mucosal edema and ulceration of the bowel

Chron's Disease

Match the anatomic part with the correct name.

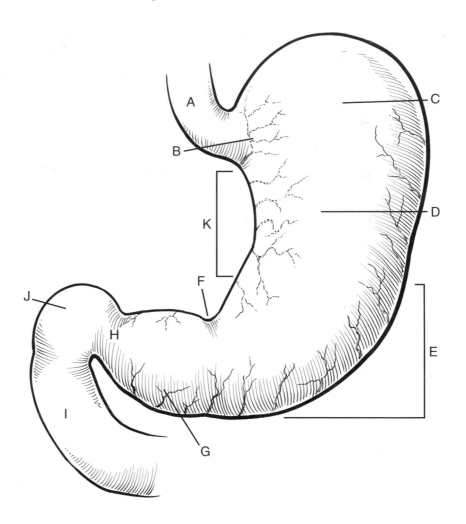

1. _N_ cecum

2. _A_ esophagus

3. _J_ duodenal bulb

4. _k_ lesser curvature

5. _C_ fundus

6. _U_ rectum

7. _K_ transverse colon

8. _V_ anus

9. _i_ duodenum

10. _M_ appendix

11. _P_ hepatic flexure

12. _L_ ileum

13. _f_ incisura

14. _B_ cardiac orifice

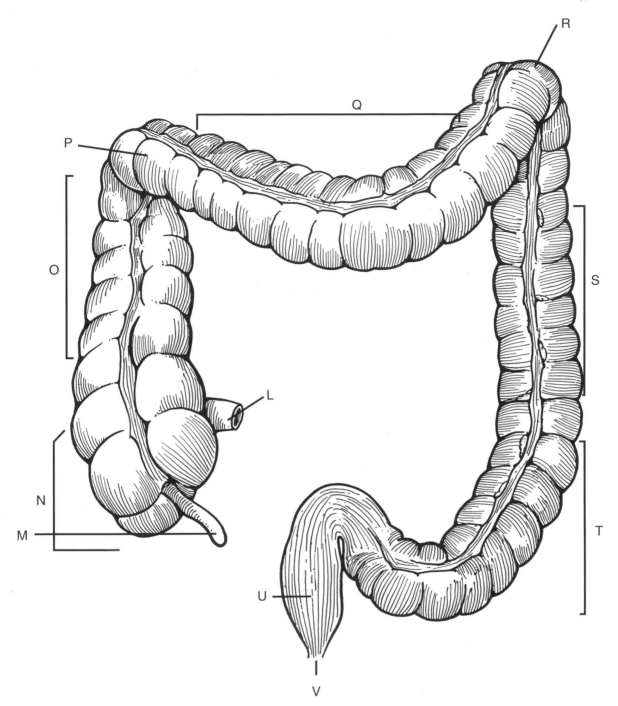

15. _R_ splenic flexure

16. _S_ descending colon

17. _E_ greater curvature

18. _D_ body

19. _D_ ascending colon

20. _G_ pylorus

21. _H_ pyloric channel

22. _T_ sigmoid

CHAPTER V SELF-TEST

There are 50 possible points on this self-test. Score it against the answers found in the exercises. A score of 47 points or higher indicates mastery and retention of this material.

Complete the blanks in the following statements.

1. The radiograph shows distended loops of bowel in the central portion of the

   film in what type of obstruction? _____

2. The pathologic condition in which the wall of the gallbladder is calcified

   is _____ .

3. Name the most frequent site of gastric ulcers.

   _____

4. A condition wherein the bowel twists over onto itself is called

   _____ .

5. What procedure uses barium and air to study the duodenum?

   _____

6. The patient must perform what maneuver to demonstrate gastric reflux into

   the esophagus? _____

7. Name the two categories of esophageal diverticula.

   _____   _____

8. Malignant tumors of the esophagus demonstrate a definite division between normal tissue and tumor. This division is termed

   _____ .

9. What type of ulcer produces the classic radiographic appearance of a

   "cloverleaf"? _____

10. Name two types of bezoars.

    _____   _____

11. Name the congenital diverticulum that represents the persistence of the yolk

    sac. _____

12. A passageway between the trachea and the esophagus is known as

    a _____ .

13. What disease is due to reflux esophagitis, which causes

    ulcerations? _____

14. Which portion of the digestive tract carries out the processes of digestion and

    absorption? _____

15. What condition is due to taking too many laxatives for too long a period of

    time? _____

Mark the statements "T" for true or "F" for false.

_T_ 16. A pharyngeal pouch can become so large as to be outwardly discernible.

_T_ 17. A congenital lack of development of the esophagus at any point is known as atresia.

_F_ 18. A 40-year-old patient who has difficulty swallowing is tested for esophageal varices. *Carcinoma*

_T_ 19. Pleural effusion can be seen on a patient who has experienced spontaneous rupture of the esophagus.

_F_ 20. The taenia coli can be seen on the radiograph and demarcates the junction of the two parts of the small bowel. *ligament of Treitz*

_T_ 21. CT and ultrasonography are useful modalities for demonstrating metastases of abdominal viscera.

_F_ 22. When a portion of the stomach slides above the diaphragm, leaving the gastroesophageal junction in place, the patient is said to have a sliding hernia. *Rolling*

_T_ 23. Hirschsprung disease is caused by the congenital absence of neurons in the colon, which prevents peristalsis.

_T_ 24. A water siphonage test is used to help determine reflux esophagitis.

_F_ 25. "Shelving" is demonstrated in ~~pyloric stenosis.~~ *esophageal carcinoma*

_F_ 26. ~~Pulsion~~ *Traction* diverticula of the esophagus have a distinctive triangular shape.

_F_ 27. The greatest amount of digestion occurs in the ~~stomach.~~ *small bowel*

Circle the letter in front of the correct answer.

28. What condition is present when large amounts of air can be seen in dilated loops of small and large bowel?
    (A) paralytic ileus
    B. localized ileus
    C. colonic ileus
    D. ischemic ileus

29. What disease shows the "string sign"?
    (A) regional enteritis
    B. Zollinger-Ellison disease
    C. esophagel varices
    D. paralytic ileus

30. The condition of one part of the bowel telescoping into another portion is known as
    A. intussusception
    B. volvulus
    C. ileus
    D. obstruction

31. Obstruction of the body of the stomach causes a sign known as
    A. "figure 8"
    B. "thumbprint"
    C. "hourglass"
    D. "leather bottle"

32. The stepladder sign is indicative of
    A. regional enteritis
    B. parasitic small bowel
    C. small bowel obstruction
    D. ulcerative colitis

33. Portal venous hypertension can result in
    A. hiatal hernia
    B. gastric ulcers
    C. esophageal varices
    D. prolapse of gastric mucosa

34. What radiograph is done to see a displaced stomach owing to retroperitoneal adenopathy?
    A. RAO
    B. LPO
    C. Lateral
    D. PA

35. Outpouchings along the walls of the bowel lumen are termed
    A. ulcers
    B. diverticula
    C. duodenal ulcer
    D. peritoneal ulcer

36. Annular carcinoma of the colon shows the classic appearance of
    A. apple-core
    B. ground glass
    C. eggshell
    D. bird's beak

37. Which type of adenocarcinoma causes the leather bottle stomach syndrome?
    A. papillary
    B. ulcerating
    C. infiltrating
    D. fungating

Match each of the following with the correct definition by placing the letter of the answer in the space provided. Each question has only one correct answer.

A. Crohn's disease

B. achalasia

C. corkscrew esophagus

D. intussusception

E. Hirschsprung disease

F. esophageal varices

G. esophageal web

H. cathartic colon

 I. pneumatosis

J. adenocarcinoma of the colon

K. spastic colon

L. pseudotumors

M. pylorospasm

N. hiatal hernia

O. Zollinger-Ellison

P. ulcerative colitis

Q. ischemic colitis

R. sprue

S. gastritis

T. trichobezoar

U. prolapse

38. _B_ shows the "rat tail" appearance

achalasia

39. _R_ also known as celiac disease

Sprue

40. _R_ shows the moulage sign

Sprue

41. _I_ air in the bowel wall

pneumatosis

42. _A_ condition that leaves "skipped areas" of normal bowel

Chron's disease

43. _A_ radiograph demonstrates a cobblestone appearance owing to mucosal edema and ulceration of the bowel

Chron's disease

44. _F_ classic appearance of rosary beads

esophageal varices

45. _P_ pseudopolyps are seen with this condition

ulcerative colitis

46. _O_ most common cause of gastric fold thickening in the fundus of the stomach

Zollinger-Elleson

47. _E_ 80% of the patients with this disease are males and exhibit failure to thrive and constipation

Hirschsprung disease

48. _T_ foreign body mass such as hair in the stomach

trichobezoar

49. _P_ has the typical sign of a lead-pipe appearance

ulcerative colitis

50. _N_ when the abdominal viscera moves through a defect in the diaphragm

hiatal hernia

Urinary System

Rationale

Trauma to the abdomen owing to high-speed automobile accidents, atheletic injuries, or gunshot and knife wounds may damage the kidneys. Because the kidneys are responsible for maintaining homeostasis, injury of the kidneys may cause waste to accumulate. Diagnostic radiographic films are an important means for detecting the presence of an injury, evaluating the nature and extent of such injuries, and determining the necessity for immediate lifesaving surgery.

In addition to those injuries of an emergency nature, those patients with a kidney stone are generally in severe pain. Many of them have been given pain medication in the emergency room that causes them to be drowsy and unresponsive. In these instances, the radiographer must be especially alert to the patient's possible allergic reaction to the injected contrast medium. If the patient has a stone that is obstructing a ureter, there may be the additional danger of hydronephrosis.

Renal disorders are also diagnosed with radiographic techniques. Many radiographs must be taken at timed intervals to evaluate the functioning ability of the kidneys. It is the responsibility of the radiographer to evaluate properly the initial "scout" film so that precious time is not lost repositioning the patient or adjusting the techical factors.

Although CT and ultrasound are being used more often, the role of the diagnostic radiographer is still essential to producing quality radiographs that help provide the physician with the information necessary to make a diagnosis.

Objectives

1. (   )   Identify the following from a cross-sectional drawing of the kidney: capsule, cortex, columns of Bertini, medulla, minor and major calyces, and renal pelvis.

2. (   )   List the three functions of the kidneys.

3. (   )   Explain why the kidneys are essential to life.

4. (   )   Name the two types of intravenous pyelograms described in the text.

5. (   )   List two types of cystography.

6. Define the following:

   (   )   retrograde urethrography   (   )   percutaneous antegrade pyelography
   (   )   retrograde pyelography   (   )   percutaneous nephrostomy

7. (   )   Name two types of renal nuclear medicine studies.

8. Define the following terms:

   (   )   oliguria   (   )   hematuria
   (   )   polyuria   (   )   uremia
   (   )   anuria   (   )   cystitis
   (   )   retention   (   )   pyelitis

9. Describe the following congenital anomalies:

( ) double collecting system   ( ) polycystic kidneys
( ) horseshoe   ( ) hypoplasia
( ) crossed ectopy   ( ) hyperplasia
( ) nephroptosis   ( ) renal ectopia

10. ( ) Explain glomerulonephritis.

11. ( ) Describe the radiographic appearance of ureteroceles.

12. ( ) Describe how hydronephrosis occurs and how it appears on the radiograph.

13. ( ) Explain how renal artery stenosis causes elevated blood pressure.

14. ( ) Define acute and chronic pyelonephritis.

15. ( ) Describe staghorn calculus and nephrocalcinosis.

16. ( ) Explain why large doses of contrast agents are necessary to visualize the parenchyma of the kidney in renal failure.

17. ( ) Describe hypernephromas and nephroblastomas.

EXERCISE VI-1

Complete the blanks in the following statements.

1. Reflux of urine from the bladder into the ureters is due

to _incompetent ureteral valve_

2. The urinary bladder has three openings connected by a wall of muscle. This

area is called the _trigone_ .

3. What are two laboratory values that indicate renal disease?

BUN   _CREATININE_

4. Lateral and inferior displacement of the right kidney is indicative of a mass in one of three areas. Name them.

pancreas _r. adrenal_

duodenum

5. What is the functioning unit of the

kidney? _nephron_

6. Name the four functions of the kidney?

produce urine _regulate fluid in blood_

secrete urine _regulate electrolytes_

7. What is the name of the examination done to evaluate stress incontinence in

women? _bead chain cystogram_

8. In the presence of renal artery stenosis, the kidney releases an enzyme that causes vasoconstriction. What is that enzyme?

renin

9. Which type of intravenous pyelogram is routinely performed when the patient is suspected or known to have hypertension?

hypertensive intravenous pyelogram

10. Congenital absence of a kidney is known

as _renal agenesis_ .

11. Congenital fusion of the lower poles of the kidneys is known

as _horshoe_ .

*12. Name the five portions of renal anatomy that constitute the renal pedicle.

renal artery   _lymph tissue_

renal vein   _renal pelvis_

nerves

13. What term denotes inflammation of the renal

pelvis? _pyelitis_

14. What is the most common congenital anomaly of the urinary

system? _duplication_

15. What is the most common cause of enlarged

kidneys? _polycystic renal disease_

EXERCISE VI-2

Look AND
Get RIGHT
ANSWERS

Mark the following statements "T" for true or "F" for false. If it is a false statement, reword it to make it true by changing the incorrect portions.

_F_   1. IVPs are done ~~for establishing normal anatomic patterns~~. to locate masses abnormalities (laboratory values, calculi

_T_   2. Nephrocalcinosis is the condition of having multiple minute calcifications throughout the kidney.

_F_   3. The ~~renal pedicle~~ is made up of the pyramids, collecting tubules, and papillae. medulla

_T_   4. The nephron consists partly of the glomerulus, which is surrounded by Bowman capsule.

_F_   5. ESWL uses ~~ultrasonography~~ to position the patient over the electrode. floroscopy

_T_   6. Duplication, or bifid collecting systems, is a congenital disorder.

_T_   7. The large majority of urinary tract infections are caused by bacteria.

_T_ 8. Ureteroceles can give the appearance of being reduced by the pressure of urine in the bladder.

_F_ 9. The nephron of the kidney is found in the ~~medulla~~ cortex.

_T_ 10. Nephrosis is the tubular degeneration of a renal nephron.

_T_ 11. Bifid collecting systems are considered an incidental finding on an IVP.

_F_ 12. Ureteroceles are dilated portions of the ureter located ~~within the renal pelvis~~ in the bladder.

_T_ 13. Hypertension is the result of a narrowing of one or more renal arteries.

_F_ 14. A ~~urinalysis~~ BUN TEST is most important in the diagnosis of renal disease.

_T_ 15. The renal pelvis is located both within and without the kidney.

EXERCISE VI-3

Circle the letter in front of the correct answer.

1. Which examination is done by inserting a catheter into the renal pelvis from the posterior lateral aspect and injecting contrast material?
   A. PAP
   B. PTC
   C. ERCP
   D. ESWL

2. Which examination is done by inserting a catheter through the bladder into the ureter and next to the renal pelvis and then injecting contrast material?
   A. retrograde urethrography
   B. retrograde pyelography
   C. retrograde cystography
   D. antegrade pyelography

3. Which of the following is nicknamed "cobra head" because of its radiographic appearance?
   A. bladder diverticula
   B. hypertrophic trabeculation
   C. ureterocele
   D. Grawitz tumor

4. Which is a malignant neoplasm of the kidney occurring in children?
   A. Grawitz tumor
   B. Wilms tumor
   C. neuroblastoma
   D. adenocarcinoma

5. What condition causes the notched appearance that an enlarged prostate gives to the bladder?
   A. nephrocalcinosis
   B. hydronephrosis
   C. hypertrophic trabeculation
   D. nephrosis

6. A kidney condition that occurs secondarily to inflammation caused by immuno-logic factors is
   A. pyelonephritis
   B. cystitis
   C. glomerulonephritis
   D. nephrolithiasis

7. Which of the following means "floating kidney"?
   A. nephroptosis
   B. renal ectopia
   C. nephrocalcinosis
   D. pelvic kidney

8. Which one of the following examinations is performed by intravenous injection of the contrast medium?
   A. retrograde urography
   B. renal arteriography
   C. percutaneous antegrade pyelography
   D. nephrography

9. What examination is done to see if a transplanted kidney is functioning properly?
   A. dynamic renogram
   B. architectural renal scan
   C. ultrasonography
   D. CT

10. Blood in the urine is termed
    A. uremia
    B. hematuria
    C. anuria
    D. oliguria

11. Which of the following is common in women and is caused by bacteria?
    A. cystitis
    B. hematuria
    C. polycystic kidneys
    D. nephroptosis

12. Diminution in the amount of urine that is being passed is termed
    A. anuria
    B. polyuria
    C. oliguria
    D. hematuria

13. How long does it take before injected contrast material reaches its greatest level of concentration in the renal collecting system?
    A. 1 minute
    B. 5 minutes
    C. 15 minutes
    D. 30 minutes

14. What is the first portion of the excretory system to be shown by the IVP?
    A. medulla
    B. calyces
    C. renal pelvis
    D. ureter

15. Filtration of waste materials from the blood takes place in the
    A. tubules
    B. Bowman capsule
    C. glomerulus
    D. papilla

EXERCISE VI-4

Match each of the following with the correct definition by placing the letter of the answer in the space provided. Each question has only one correct answer.

A. glomerulonephritis

B. hydronephrosis

C. nephrosis

D. pyelonephritis

E. renal calculi

F. polycystic renal disease

G. horseshoe kidney

H. crossed ectopy

I. renal agenesis

J. renal ectopia

K. hyperplasia

L. prostatic hypertrophy

1. _D_ this condition is associated with blunted calyces and probable dilation of the collecting system   *pyelonephritis*

2. _K_ this condition is associated with renal agenesis on one side
hyperplasia

3. _F_ this disease eventually replaces all renal tissue; the kidney is lobulated and enlarged
polycystic renal diease

4. _C_ tubular degeneration of the collecting tubules
nephrosis

5. _H_ one kidney is located across the midline on the same side as the other
cross ectopy

6. _B_ shows sharp calyces along with dilation of the collecting system
hydronephrosis

7. _J_ associated with a congenitally short ureter
renal ectopia

8. _F_ presents as multiple cysts around the age of 30
polycustic renal diease

9. _A_ also known as Bright disease
glomerulonephritis

10. _I_ absence of one kidney
renal agenesis

11. _A_ inflammatory disease of the glomeruli
glomerulonephritis

12. _J_ misplaced kidneys usually found in the pelvis
renal ectopia

13. _A_ most common cause of small kidneys
glomerulonephritis

14. _L_ prostate gland enlargement
prostatic hypertrophy

15. _A_ patient exhibits edema of the face and ankles
glomerulonephritis

16. _D_ caused by *E. coli* bacteria
pyelonephritis

17. _E_ form from urine, which contains crystalline materials
renal calculi

18. _H_ fusion of both kidneys on one side of the body
cross ectopy

19. _B_ result of some obstruction in the renal pelvis or ureter
hydronephrosis

20. _E_ usually asymptomatic until they begin to descend through the ureters
renal calculi

Match each of the following with the correct definition by placing the letter of the answer in the space provided. Each question has only one correct answer.

A. retrograde urethrography

B. renal angiography

C. PAP

D. nephrography

E. retrograde pyelography

F. ESWL

G. cystogram

H. voiding cystogram

I. renogram

J. IVP

K. nephrotomography

L. ultrasonography

1. _D_ kidney study in which the film is taken immediately after injection of the contrast agent to show the blush of the cortex

   nephography

2. _A_ study showing the urethra on males without the patient voiding

   retrograde urethrography

3. _B_ study done to demonstrate the vascularity of the renal system

   renal angiography

4. _K_ demonstrates delayed filling of the kidneys

   nephrotomography

5. _J_ a radiographic test of the function of a kidney

   IVP

6. _E_ done by inserting a catheter as close to the pelvis of the kidney as possible and injecting contrast material

   retrograde pyelography

7. _G_ done by inserting a catheter into the bladder

   cystogram

8. _I_ a nuclear medicine study of the renal area

   renogram

9. _E_ done by inserting a catheter into the ureter to study the renal system

   retrograde pyelography

10. _L_ done for patients who are allergic to contrast media or who have an elevated blood urea nitrogen level

    ultrasonography?

11. _F_ uses focused shock waves to disintegrate renal stones

    ESWL

12. _L_ best performed on patients who are pregnant and should not be subjected to radiation

    ultrasonography

13. _H_ the patient voids during the filming of this study

    voiding cystogram

14. _B_ assessment of renal artery stenosis

    renal angiography

15. _C_ direct puncture of the renal pelvis through the posterior lateral aspect of the patient

    PAP

CHAPTER VI SELF-TEST

There are 50 possible points on this self-test. Score it against the answers found in the exercises. A score of 47 points or higher indicates mastery and retention of this material.

Complete the blanks in the following statements.

1. What is the functioning unit of the

   kidney? _nephron_____

2. Congenital absence of a kidney is known

   as _renal agenesis_____.

3. What is inflammation of the renal pelvis termed?

   _pyelitis_____

4. Lateral and inferior displacement of the right kidney is indicative of a mass in one of three areas. Name them.

   _pancreas_____   _r. adrenal_____

   _duodenum_____

5. What is the most common cause of enlarged

   kidneys? _polycystic renal disease_

6. Which type of intravenous pyelogram is routinely performed when the patient is suspected or known to have hypertension?

   hypertensive intravenous pyelogram

7. What are two laboratory values that indicate renal disease?

   _BUN_____   _CREATININE_____

8. Congenital fusion of the lower poles of the kidneys is known

   horse shoe

   as ___horshoe___ .

9. What is the most common congenital anomaly of the urinary

   system? ___duplication___

Mark the following statements "T" for true and "F" for false.

___F___ 10. Ureteroceles are dilated portions of the ureter located within the ~~renal pelvis~~. *bladder*

___T___ 11. Duplication, or bifid collecting systems, is a congenital disorder.

___T___ 12. Nephrocalcinosis is the condition of having multiple minute calcifications throughout the kidney.

___F___ 13. ESWL uses ~~ultrasonography~~ *flouroscopy* to position the patient over the electrode.

___T___ 14. Hypertension is the result of a narrowing of one or more renal arteries.

___T___ 15. Nephrosis is the tubular degeneration of a renal nephron.

___F___ 16. IVPs are done for ~~establishing normal anatomic patterns~~.

___T___ 17. Ureteroceles can give the appearance of being reduced by the pressure of urine in the bladder.

___T___ 18. Bifid collecting systems are considered an incidental finding on an IVP.

Circle the letter in front of the correct answer.

19. What condition causes the notched appearance that an enlarged prostate gives to the bladder?
    A. nephrocalcinosis
    B. hydronephrosis
    C. hypertrophic trabeculation
    D. nephrosis

20. Which examination is done by inserting a catheter into the renal pelvis from the posterior lateral aspect and injecting contrast material?
    A. PAP
    B. PTC
    C. ERCP
    D. ESWL

21. Which of the following is common in women and is caused by bacteria?
    A. cystitis
    B. hematuria
    C. polycystic kidneys
    D. nephroptosis

22. Which of the following is nicknamed "cobra head" because of its radiographic appearance?
    A. bladder diverticula
    B. hypertrophic trabeculation
    C. ureterocele
    D. Grawitz tumor

23. How long does it take before injected contrast material reaches its greatest level of concentration in the renal collecting system?
    A. 1 minute
    B. 5 minutes
    C. 15 minutes
    D. 30 minutes

24. Which one of the following examinations is performed by intravenous injection of the contrast medium?
    A. retrograde urography
    B. renal arteriography
    C. percutaneous antegrade pyelography
    D. nephrography

25. Which examination is done by inserting a catheter through the bladder into the ureter and next to the renal pelvis and then injecting contrast material?
    A. retrograde urethrography
    B. retrograde pyelography
    C. retrograde cystography
    D. antegrade pyelography

26. Diminution in the amount of urine that is being passed is termed
    A. anuria
    B. polyuria
    C. oliguria
    D. hematuria

27. Which of the following means "floating kidney"?
    A. nephroptosis
    B. renal ectopia
    C. nephrocalcinosis
    D. pelvic kidney

28. Blood in the urine is termed
    A. uremia
    B. hematuria
    C. anuria
    D. oliguria

29. What is the first portion of the excretory system to be shown by the IVP?
    A. medulla
    (B) calyces
    C. renal pelvis
    D. ureter

Match each of the following with the correct definition by placing the letter of the answer in the space provided. Each question has only one correct answer.

A. glomerulonephritis

B. hydronephrosis

C. nephrosis

D. pyelonephritis

E. renal calculi

F. polycystic renal disease

G. horseshoe kidney

H. crossed ectopy

I. renal agenesis

J. renal ectopia

K. hyperplasia

L. prostatic hypertrophy

30. __F__ presents as multiple cysts around the age of 30

polycystic renal disease

31. __H__ one kidney is located across the midline on the same side as the other

crossed ectopy

32. __J__ misplaced kidneys usually found in the pelvis

renal ectopia

33. __K__ condition associated with renal agenesis on one side

hyperplasia

34. __A__ most common cause of small kidneys

35. __J__ associated with a congenitally short ureter

36. __A__ patient exhibits edema of the face and ankles

glomerulonephritis

37. __F__ this disease eventually replaces all renal tissue; the kidney is lobulated and enlarged

38. __L__ prostate gland enlargement

prostatic hypertophy

39. __A__ also known as Bright disease

glomerulenephritis

40. __I__ absence of one kidney

renal agenesis

A. retrograde urethrography

B. renal angiography

C. PAP

D. nephrography

E. retrograde pyelography

F. ESWL

G. cystogram

H. voiding cystogram

I. ultrasonography

J. IVP

41. _B_ assessment of renal artery stenosis

42. _I_ done for patients who are allergic to contrast media or who have an elevated blood urea nitrogen level

43. _G_ done by inserting a catheter into the bladder

44. _A_ study showing the urethra on males without the patient voiding

45. _E_ done by inserting a catheter as close to the pelvis of the kidney as possible and injecting contrast material

46. _D_ kidney study in which the film is taken immediately after injection of the contrast medium to show the blush of the cortex

47. _C_ direct puncture of the renal pelvis through the posterior lateral aspect of the patient

48. _F_ uses focused shock waves to disintegrate renal stones

49. _B_ study done to demonstrate the vascularity of the renal system

50. _E_ done by inserting a catheter into the ureter to study the renal system

Reproductive System

Rationale

Modern technology in the form of nonionizing ultrasound has replaced many of the once common radiographic examinations that were performed on the pregnant patient. Examinations such as x-ray pelvimetry are no longer performed.

Examinations of the female and male reproductive organs, such as hysterosalpingograms and retrograde urethrograms, are still performed. Patients undergoing these examinations are often embarrassed or uncomfortable with a physician they are unfamiliar with and a technologist who is assisting this physician. The role of the radiographer is not only to assist the radiologist, but also to see to the comfort of the patient. Simple reassurance and a sense of empathy are often the key to helping the patient relax, thus enabling the examination to go more smoothly and involve less discomfort. Professionalism on the part of the radiographer is of the utmost importance in any radiographic examination of the reproductive system. An understanding of the possible diagnosis is an important part of professional ethics.

Objectives

1. ( ) Identify the fundus, body, and cervix of the uterus from a drawing.

2. ( ) Describe the normal and abnormal positions of the uterus.

3. ( ) Identify the testis, epididymis, and vas deferens within the scrotum from a drawing.

4. ( ) Describe a hysterosalpingogram.

5. ( ) List the congenital anomalies of the shape of the uterus.

6. ( ) Explain the condition of cryptorchidism.

7. ( ) Describe the condition of endometriosis.

8. ( ) Define pelvic inflammatory disease.

9. ( ) List the three types of fibroids.

10. ( ) Explain the difference between endometrial and cervical carcinoma.

11. ( ) Define epididymitis and gynecomastia.

12. ( ) Describe testicular torsion.

13. ( ) Explain the difference between a hydrocele and a spermatocele.

14. ( ) Describe a seminoma.

EXERCISE VII-1

Complete the blanks in the following statements.

1. Name the three parts of the uterine cavity.

fundus _cervix_

body

2. What is the normal position of the uterus called?

anteverted, anteflexed

3. Name the "cuff" that the vagina forms around the cervix.

fornix

4. Name the four parts of the female reproductive system.

vagina _ovaries_

uterus _uterine tube_

5. What is an accessory organ to the female reproductive system?

breast

6. Cystic dilation of the epididymis is known as

spermatocele.

7. Hydronephrosis is seen on the intravenous pyelogram in what type of female

carcinoma? _Cervical_

8. The basic structural unit of the breast is the

_____ lobule _____.

9. Which glands secrete an alkaline fluid that protects the sperm from vaginal fluid? _Cowper (bulbourethral)_

10. Name the three phases of the menstrual cycle.

proliferative   _menstrual_

secretory

11. The process of the lobules of the breast decreasing in size and number is called _involution_.

12. The formation of sperm is known as

Spermatogenesis.

13. What hormone is responsible for adult male sexual behavior?

testosterone

14. What is the major disadvantage to the use of water-soluble contrast media in hysterosalpingograms?

produces pain

15. Name the two routine positions in mammography.

craniocaudal   _medial lateral oblique_

16. What three functions do cones in mammography serve?

prevents scatters   makes positioning better

helps with Compression

17. The uterus is made from paired ducts that fuse to become the uterus and the uterine tubes. These are known as

mullerian ducts .

18. What condition exists when there is a septum extending through the normal uterine body dividing it into two complete compartments?

septate

19. Identify the anatomic parts indicated.

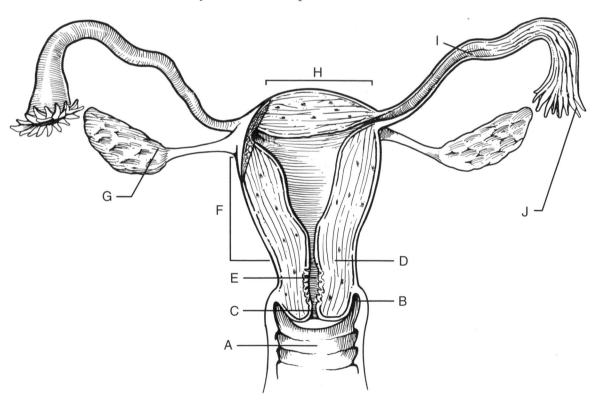

A. vagina

B. fornix

C. external os

D. cervix

E. internal os

F. body

G. ovary

H. fundus

I. uterine tube

J. fimbre

20. Identify the abnormal uterine positions indicated.

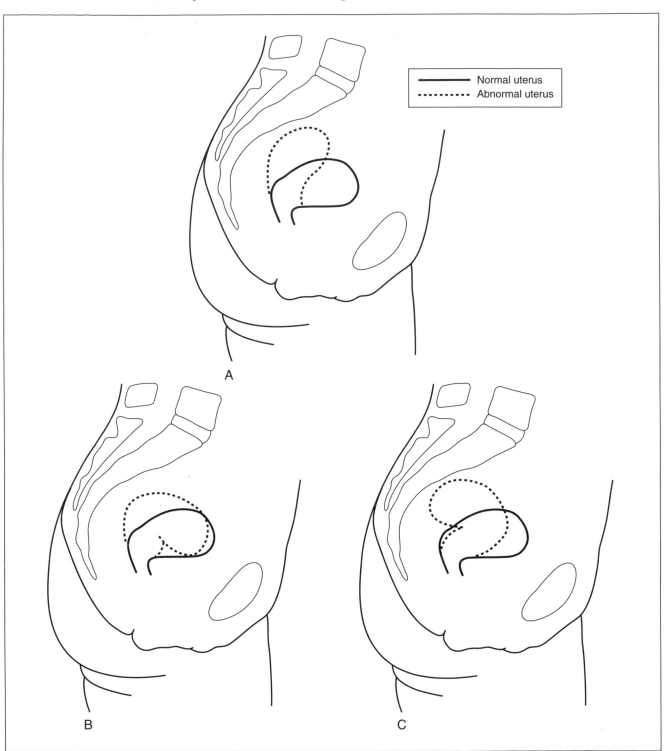

β A. <u>retroversion</u>

A B. <u>antiflexion</u>

C. <u>retroflexion</u>

EXERCISE VII-2

Mark the following statements "T" for true or "F" for false. If it is a false statement, reword it to make it true by changing the incorrect portions.

_F_ 1. Pyosalpinx may result if a ~~tubal ovarian abscess~~ _PID_ is left untreated.

_T_ 2. A didelphic uterus is rare.

_T_ 3. If there is a uterine anomaly, there is likely to be renal agenesis on that side as well.

_T_ 4. Leiomyoma is another name for a fibroid.

_F_ 5. Adenomyosis usually coexists with ~~myomas~~ _endometriosis_.

_F_ 6. Fifty percent to 60 percent of pelvic inflammatory disease is caused by ~~IUDs~~ _veneral diseases_.

_T_ 7. National Cancer Institute guidelines state that women 50 years and older should have a yearly mammogram.

_F_ 8. An ~~intravenous pyelogram~~ _endometral carcinoma_ shows the bladder indented by an enlarged uterus with cervical carcinoma.

_T_ 9. The most common cause of death in patients with cervical carcinoma is impaired renal function.

_T_ 10. Women who delay their first pregnancy tend to have a higher relative risk of breast cancer than women who have a pregnancy at age 17.

_F_ 11. Young, nulligrava women have ~~fat infiltration of the~~ _dense_ breasts.

_F_ 12. ~~Benign~~ _Malignant tumors_ breast lesions appear as sandlike grains of calcifications on the mammogram.

_F_ 13. Dedicated mammographic units have a ~~tungsten~~ _molybdenum_ target similar to a regular radiographic unit.

_F_ 14. ~~Adenomyosis~~ _Endometriosis_ is the growth of endometrial tissue outside the uterus.

_T_ 15. Severe pain with the menstrual period is known as dysmenorrhea.

_T_ 16. The most common invasive gynecologic malignancy of the uterus is endometrial carcinoma.

_F_ 17. The condition of undescended testis is known as ~~orchiopexy~~ _criptochidism_.

_T_ 18. Enlargement of the male breast is known as gynecomastia.

_T_ 19. Doppler ultrasound can be used to differentiate between testicular torsion and epididymitis.

_T_ 20. The characteristic "fish hook" appearance of the distal ureters is demonstrated on the intravenous pyelogram with prostatic hyperplasia.

EXERCISE VII-3

Circle the letter in front of the correct answer.

1. Which of the following concerning fibroids is *not* true?
   A. can cause abortion
   B. thrive on estrogen
   C. usually menopausal women have them
   D. can prevent delivery of fetus

2. If contrast material spills into the pelvis and outlines the small bowel loops during hysterosalpingography, one may assume
   A. an error in technique
   B. too much contrast material has been used
   C. the tubes are patent
   D. the bowel is abnormal

3. The absence of a uterus is known as
   A. uterine aplasia
   B. didelphic uterus
   C. arcuate uterus
   D. bicornate bicollic uterus

4. Where is the fornix located?
   A. external os
   B. internal os
   C. corpus of uterus
   D. fundus

5. What word does *not* belong?
   A. fimbriae
   B. infundibulum
   C. isthmus
   D. intramural

6. Which type of fibroid is mostly pedunculated?
   A. subserous
   B. intramural
   C. submucosal
   D. leiomyoma

7. Which is *not* a contraindication for doing a hysterosalpingogram?
   A. pelvic inflammatory disease
   B. vaginal infection
   C. pregnancy
   D. infertility

8. All are pieces of equipment used in hysteropsalpingograms *except*
   A. endoscope
   B. tenaculum
   C. speculum
   D. cannula

9. What type of breast tissue enhances radiographic visibility of possible masses?
   A. dense
   B. fatty
   C. mixed
   D. cystic

10. Diagnostic indications for hysterosalpingograms include all of the following *except*
    A. habitual spontaneous abortions
    B. amenorrhea
    C. cervical infection
    D. bleeding between menstrual periods

11. How much contrast medium is needed to fill the uterus?
    A. 2 mL
    B. 4 mL
    C. 8 mL
    D. 100 mL

12. Which is the most important function of mammography?
    A. to show the size of a mass
    B. reveal calcifications
    C. early detection and diagnosis of breast cancer
    D. demonstrate nipple inversion

13. Normal kV range in mammography is
    A. 4–16
    B. 25–30
    C. 45–55
    D. 80–125

14. Which study is done to evaluate testicular mass blood flow?
    A. CT
    B. hysterosalpingogram
    C. angiography
    D. Doppler ultrasonography

15. What term is used to denote a uterus wherein the fundus and body are posterior to the cervix?
    A. anteflexion
    B. retroflexed
    C. retroversion
    D. anteversion

EXERCISE VII-4

Match each of the following with the correct definition by placing the letter of the answer in the space provided. Each question has only one correct answer.

A. pelvic inflammatory disease

B. tubal ovarian abscess

C. fibroid

D. bicornate uterus

E. uterine aplasia

F. unicornuate uterus

G. arcuate uterus

H. didelphic uterus

I. bicornate bicollic

J. adenomyosis

K. endometriosis

L. pyosalpinx

M. ovarian cystadenoma

N. polycystic ovaries

O. dermoid cysts

P. fibroadenoma

Q. breast carcinoma

R. hydrocele

S. prostate carcinoma

T. endometrial carcinoma

1. __C__ most common benign tumor of the uterus = fibroid

2. __K__ usually occurs in nulliparous women over age 30
   endometriosis

3. __K__ also known as a chocolate cyst
   endometriosis

4. __G__ nonfusion of the müllerian ducts beginning at the level of the fundus
   arcuate uterus

5. __H__ complete duplication of the reproductive organs
   didelphic uterus

6. __D__ common anomaly of having one vagina, one cervix, one body, but two fundi
   bicornate uterus

7. __J__ the ingrowth of endometrium
   adenomyosis

8. __L__ pus in the uterine tube
   pyosalpinx

9. __F__ one half of a uterine cavity owing to formation of only one müllerian duct
   unicornate uterus

10. __G__ most common congenital anomaly of the female reproductive system
    arcuate uterus

11. __F__ an elongated uterus with a single uterine tube

unicornuate uterus

12. __O__ often contain hair, fat, bone, or teeth

~~fibroid~~ *dermoid cyst*

13. __N__ enlarged ovaries with multiple cysts and associated with Stein-Leventhal syndrome

polycystic ovaries

14. __P__ most common benign breast mass

fibroadenoma

15. __Q__ has the highest mortality rate of all cancers in females

breast carcinoma

16. __S__ skeletal metastases occur in approximately 75% of all cases

prostate carcinoma

17. __M__ most common benign tumor of the ovary

ovarian cystadenoma

18. __O__ masses arising from unfertilized ova

dermoid cyst

19. __C__ a solid benign tumor of the uterus that tends to shrink after menopause

20. __B__ pyosalpinx eventually leads to this

Match the anatomic part with the correct name.

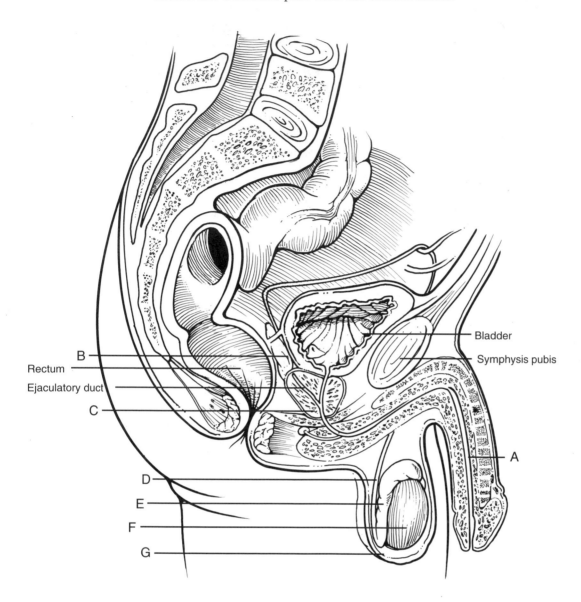

Bladder

Symphysis pubis

B

Rectum

Ejaculatory duct

C

A

D

E

F

G

21. _C_ prostate

22. _E_ epididymis

23. _D_ vas deferens

24. _B_ seminal vesicle

25. _A_ urethra

26. _F_ testicle

27. _G_ scrotum

CHAPTER VII SELF-TEST

There are 50 possible points on this self-test. Score it against the answers found in the exercises. A score of 47 points or higher indicates mastery and retention of this material.

Complete the blanks in the following statements.

1. What three functions do cones in mammography serve?

   _____   _____

   _____

2. What is the major disadvantage to the use of water-soluble contrast media in hysterosalpingograms?

   _pain_____

3. What is the normal position of the uterus called?

   _antiflex/anteverted_____

4. Cystic dilation of the epididymis is known as

   _spermatocele_____.

5. The formation of sperm is known as

   _spermagenesis_____.

6. Name the "cuff" that the vagina forms around the cervix.

    fornix

7. The uterus is made from paired ducts that fuse to become the uterus and the uterine tubes. These are known as

    mullerian .

8. What hormone is responsible for adult male sexual behavior?

    _____

9. Hydronephrosis is seen on the intravenous pyelogram in what type of carcinoma in females?

    cervical

10. What condition exists when there is a septum extending through the normal uterine body dividing it into two complete compartments?

    _____

11. Which glands secrete an alkaline fluid that protects the sperm from vaginal fluid?

    Cowpers

12. Name the two routine positions in mammography.

    _____   _____

Mark the following statements "T" for true or "F" for false.

_F_   *Endometriosis*
    13. ~~Adenomyosis~~ usually coexists with myomas.

_T_   14. National Cancer Institute guidelines state that women 50 years and older should have a yearly mammogram.

_T_ _____ 15. The most common cause of death in patients with cervical carcinoma is impaired renal function.

_T_ _____ 16. Severe pain with the menstrual period is known as dysmenorrhea.

_F_ _____ *Malignant* 17. ~~Benign~~ breast lesions appear as sandlike grains of calcifications on the mammogram.

_T_ _____ 18. Doppler ultrasound can be used to differentiate between testicular torsion and epididymitis.

_T_ _____ 19. A didelphic uterus is rare.

_T_ _____ 20. The most common invasive gynecologic malignancy of the uterus is endometrial carcinoma.

_T_ _____ 21. Leiomyoma is another name for a fibroid.

_F_ _____ *cryptorchism* 22. The condition of undesended testis is known as ~~orchiopexy~~.

_F_ _____ *molybdenum* 23. Dedicated mammographic units have a ~~tungsten~~ target similar to a regular radiographic unit.

_F_ _____ 24. An intravenous pyelogram shows the bladder indented by an enlarged uterus with ~~cervical~~ carcinoma.
endometrial

_F_ _____ 25. Adenomyosis is the growth of endometrial tissue outside the uterus.

_T_ _____ 26. The characteristic "fish hook" appearance of the distal ureters is demonstrated on the intravenous pyelogram with prostatic hyperplasia.

Circle the letter in front of the correct answer.

27. Which is *not* a contraindication for a hysterosalpingogram?
    A. pelvic inflammatory disease
    B. vaginal infection
    C. pregnancy
    (D.) infertility

28. Which of the following concerning fibroids is *not* true?
    A. can cause abortion
    B. thrive on estrogen
    (C.) usually menopausal women have them
    D. can prevent delivery of fetus

29. How much contrast medium is needed to fill the uterus?
    A. 2 mL
    (B.) 4 mL
    C. 8 mL
    D. 100 mL

30. All are pieces of equipment used in hysteropsalpingograms *except*
    A. endoscope
    B. tenaculum
    C. speculum
    D. cannula

31. The absence of a uterus is known as
    A. uterine aplasia
    B. didelphic uterus
    C. arcuate uterus
    D. bicornate bicollic uterus

32. Diagnostic indications for hysterosalpingograms include all of the following *except*
    A. habitual spontaneous abortions
    B. amenorrhea
    C. cervical infection
    D. bleeding between menstrual periods

33. Which type of fibroid is mostly pedunculated?
    A. subserous
    B. intramural
    C. submucosal
    D. leiomyoma

34. What type of breast tissue enhances radiographic visibility of possible masses?
    A. dense
    B. fatty
    C. mixed
    D. cystic

35. If contrast material spills into the pelvis and outlines the small bowel loops during hysterosalpingography, one may assume
    A. an error in technique
    B. too much contrast material has been used
    C. the tubes are patent
    D. the bowel is abnormal

36. Normal kV range in mammography is
    A. 4–16
    B. 25–30
    C. 45–55
    D. 80–125

37. Which study is done to evaluate testicular mass blood flow?
    A. CT
    B. hysterosalpingogram
    C. angiography
    D. Doppler ultrasonography

38. Which is the most important function of mammography?
    A. to show the size of a mass
    B. to reveal calcifications
    C. to allow early detection and diagnosis of breast cancer
    D. to demonstrate nipple inversion

STD

Syphillis — caused by a spirokete has canker sore
can be successfully treated

Gonnorhea — more silent.
women - discharge all the time
male - drip discharge
Causes PID and sterility

Male sterility
↓below 50 million

Match each of the following with the correct definition by placing the letter of the answer in the space provided. Each question has only one correct answer.

A. pelvic inflammatory disease

B. tubal ovarian abscess

C. fibroid

D. bicornate uterus

E. uterine aplasia

F. unicornuate uterus

G. arcuate uterus

H. didelphic uterus

I. bicornate bicollis

J. adenomyosis

K. endometriosis

L. pyosalpinx

M. ovarian cystadenoma

N. polycystic ovaries

O. dermoid cysts

P. fibroadenoma

Q. breast carcinoma

R. hydrocele

S. prostate carcinoma

T. endometrial carcinoma

39. __C__ a solid benign tumor of the uterus that tends to shrink after menopause

fibroid

40. __C__ most common benign tumor of the uterus

fibroid

41. __J__ the ingrowth of endometrium

adenomyosis

42. __Q__ has the highest mortality rate of all cancers in females

breast carcinoma

43. __G__ nonfusion of the müllerian ducts beginning at the level of the fundus

unicornate uterus)

44. __P__ most common benign breast mass

fibroadenoma

45. __k__ usually occurs in nulliparous women over age 30

endometriosis

46. __M__ most common benign tumor of the ovary

ovarian cystadenoma

47. __D__ common anomaly of having one vagina, one cervix, one body, but two fundi

bicornate uterus

48. __O__ often contain hair, fat, bone, or teeth

dermoid cyst

49. __S__ skeletal metastases occur in approximately 75% of all cases

prostate carcinoma)

50. __F__ one half of a uterine cavity owing to formation of only one müllerian duct

unicornate uterus)

Respiratory System

Rationale

The most common radiograph is the chest examination. As such, this radiographic examination is often the one that is performed the quickest and, sometimes, the most carelessly. The radiographer must remember that the chest is one of the most complex areas in the body. This examination is not just about the heart and lungs. The radiograph should also show the lower cervical spine area, the clavicles, perhaps even the shoulders, the diaphragm, the thoracic spine (or a portion of it), and air levels below the diaphragm.

The radiographer must take the time when viewing the finished radiographs to make sure that the apices or the cupula areas have not been clipped and that the heart has been adequately penetrated but that the lung fields are not burned out. "Hot lighting" the upper lung fields does not provide the same information that an appropriately exposed film provides. An underexposed radiograph can cause the appearance of pathology in the lungs or obscure an area of pathology that would normally be seen on a good radiograph.

Positioning of the patient must be done with sufficient care that symmetry of the clavicles is ensured and that the radiographer is satisfied that both apices are present on the film. An understanding of the pathologies that may be simulated owing to improper positioning is essential for avoiding common errors.

Proper breathing instructions should be given to the patient before positioning the patient so that he or she does not move to ask what to do. Maximum inspiration is obtained when the patient inhales, exhales, and then inhales a second time. Also, shielding of the patient should be completed before positioning so that the patient does not need to be recentered to the cassette. A well-organized technologist saves time while still providing excellent patient care.

Objectives

1. (   ) List the physiology and function of the trachea and bronchi and the respiratory system as a whole.

2. (   ) Explain the purpose of the apical lordotic view of the chest.

3. (   ) Describe the method of radiographing the lungs on inspiration and expiration.

4. (   ) Explain how the body habitus and position would affect the chest radiograph.

5. (   ) Describe a bronchogram.

6. (   ) Define laryngography.

7. (   ) Identify the use of ultrasound in imaging of the lungs.

8. (   ) Explain respiratory distress syndrome.

9. (   ) List three types of abscesses of the lungs.

10. (   ) Describe atelectasis and name at least two causes.

11. (   ) Explain the difference between bronchitis and bronchiectasis.

12. (   ) Name two types of emphysema and describe them.

13. ( ) Identify pleural effusion on upright and lateral decubitus radiographs of the chest.

14. ( ) Name five types of pneumonitis seen on radiographs.

15. ( ) Describe the appearance of lobar pneumonia.

16. ( ) Explain how aspiration pneumonia occurs.

17. ( ) List three types of pneumoconioses.

18. ( ) Describe tension pneumothorax.

19. ( ) Describe the appearance of the two types of tuberculosis.

20. ( ) Name three types of metastatic bronchogenic carcinomas.

21. ( ) List three types of mediastinal masses.

22. ( ) Explain pneumomediastinum.

EXERCISE VIII-1

Complete the blanks in the following statements.

1. Another name for the voice box is

the _larynx_ .

larynx

2. What is the name of the area of bifurcation of the

trachea? _Carina_

Carina

3. Which hilum should always appear higher on the

radiograph? _left   lingua_

left lingua

4. Name the fissure that divides the right middle lobe from the right lower

lobe. _Oblique_   _oblique_

5. Supine chest films are unacceptable because they cause the appearance of

what pathology of the heart? _congestive heart failure_

Congestive heart failure

6. Name the two categories of iodinated contrast media used in bronchograms.

aqueous (absorbed)   _oily (removed)_

aqueous (absorbed)   *oily (removed)*

7. Name the three most commonly used procedures for introduction of contrast in bronchograms.

catheter insertion   _aspiration_

percutaneous transtracheal

8. The confluence of major bronchi and vessels in each lung is called

the _hilum_ .

hilum

9. In the lung, a localized necrosis of tissue is known as

an _abscess_ .

abscess

10. Name the layers of the pleura of the lung.

visceral   _parital_

visceral   *parital*

11. What radiographic procedure is often required to confirm the diagnosis of bronchiectasis when routine chest radiographs are

inconclusive? _bronchography_

12. Name the three most common pneumoconioses. *(dust particles*

silocoisis   _berystolisis_

silocoisis   *berystolisis*

abestosis

abestosis

13. What is the hereditary disease in which thick mucus is secreted and affects the

lungs? _cyptic fibrosis_

cyptic fibrosis

14. The functional unit for gas exchange in the lungs is

the _alveoli_ .

alveoli

[handwritten margin notes: anterior / posterior / middle / superior]

[handwritten margin notes: pulmonary embolism / hampton hump]

15. Name the four divisions of the mediastinum that are used when defining pathology.

[handwritten: superior / super _____   *middle* _____]

[handwritten: anterior _____   *posterior* _____]

16. When a characteristic inverted wedge-shaped opacity of the lung is seen on a radiograph, it may indicate the presence of

a *[handwritten: pulmonary embolism]* _____
[handwritten: pulmonary embolism]

17. When areas of fluid consolidation collapse and oppose each other, they cause the bronchi to become visible. This is known as what radiographic

sign? *[handwritten: air bronchogram]* _____
[handwritten: air bronchogram]

18. With what pathology is a lung edge

seen? *[handwritten: pneumothorax]* _____
[handwritten: pneumothorax]

19. Permanent dilation of the bronchi is known

as *[handwritten: bronchiectasis]* _____.
[handwritten: bronchiectasis]

20. Obstruction of a bronchus is the most common cause

of *[handwritten: atelectasis atelectasis]* _____

[handwritten margin notes: No shift / carcinoma / shift]

EXERCISE VIII-2

Mark the following statements "T" for true or "F" for false. If the statement is false, reword it to make it true by changing the incorrect portions.

___*T*___ 1. Calcification in a coin lesion of the lung usually means the lesion is benign.

___*F*___ *[handwritten: COPD are interchangeble names]* 2. Emphysema is another name for atelectasis.

___*T*___ 3. Lobar pneumonia mostly involves lung alveoli of an entire lobe.

_____ 4. The pharynx is part of the respiratory and digestive systems.

_F_   5. Rotation of the patient during chest radiography may cause the appearance of ~~loss of lung volume~~. _congestive hear failure & magnification_

_T_   6. Lobar pneumonia is an acute disease caused by a bacterial organism.

_T_   7. Embolic abscess is due to an infected blood clot reaching the lung.

_F_   8. When a pneumothorax is suspected, the radiographer should take _single_ ~~double~~ exposure inhalation-exhalation films of the chest. _(↑ best)_

_T_   9. One common reason for obtaining a chest radiograph is a patient history of asthma.

_F_   10. Bronchitis is the medical term for infection of the ~~air sacs~~ _bronchi_ within the lungs. _alveoli_

_T_   11. Emphysema is incurable.

_T_   12. Pleurisy refers to an inflammation of the lining of the lungs.

_T_   13. Inhaling a peanut may cause a collapsed lung, or a portion of it.

_T_   14. Inhaling a peanut may cause an abscess of the lung.

_T_   15. Inhaling a peanut may cause aspiration pneumonia. _right bronchus_

_F_   16. Pneumonia is a term used to describe an inflammation of the ~~bronchus~~ _lung_.

_T_   17. Centrilobular emphysema is more commonly known as chronic obstructive pulmonary disease.

_T_   18. Leather lung disease is so called because the lung becomes stiff and brittle.

_T_   19. Interstitial pneumonia is also known as viral pneumonia.

_F_   20. Heart magnification is greater on a ~~PA~~ _AP_ chest radiograph than it is on an ~~AP~~ _PA_ radiograph.

EXERCISE VIII-3

Circle the letter in front of the correct answer.

1. An overexpanded lung can cause all of the following _except_
    A. mediastinal shift
    B. atelectasis
    C. flattened hemidiaphragm
    D. pleural effusion

2. What is the most common change seen on a routine, yearly chest radiograph?
   A. increased heart size
   B. emphysema
   C. pleurisy
   D. pericardial effusion

   increased heart size

3. Which portion of the mediastinum is not used in radiography?
   A. superior
   B. anterior
   C. middle
   D. posterior

   Superior

4. To check for deep inspiration in an adult, the diaphragm should be at which level?
   A. T-11
   B. T-8
   C. T-12
   D. sternal notch

   T-11

5. Which of the following is *not* part of the mediastinum?
   A. heart
   B. lungs
   C. trachea
   D. lymph tissue

   lungs

6. Which of the following chest pathologies would require a decrease in technique from a "normal" chest radiograph?
   A. atelectasis
   B. pneumothorax
   C. pleural effusion
   D. pneumonia

   pneumothorax

7. What is the most inferior and lateral portion of the lung called?
   A. costophrenic angle
   B. apex
   C. hilus
   D. axilla

   Costophrenic angle

8. Which of the following is responsible for air exchange?
   A. diaphragm
   B. hilus
   C. alveolus
   D. bronchus

   alveolus

9. The carina is found at the level of
   A. C-7
   B. T-2
   C. T-5
   D. T-8

   T-5

10. Anterior oblique views of the chest demonstrate all but the
    A. heart
    B. aortic arch
    C. pulmonary artery
    D. abdominal aorta

    abdominal aorta

11. If an upright chest radiograph cannot be performed, what position is used to demonstrate pleural effusion?
    A. cross table lateral
    B. transthoracic
    C. lateral decubitus
    D. Trendelenburg

    lateral decub

12. Which of the following structures can be well demonstrated on a lateral chest projection?
    A. trachea
    B. interlobar fissure
    C. bronchi
    D. mediastinum

    mediastinum

13. Patient rotation can be evaluated on a PA chest radiograph by assessing
    A. the curvature of the thoracic spine
    B. the scapula in the lung fields
    C. sternoclavicular joint asymmetry
    D. the height of the clavicles

    Sternoclavicular joint asymmetry

14. Which of the following respiratory disorders is *not* associated with chronic obstructive pulmonary disease?
    A. bronchitis
    B. emphysema
    C. tuberculosis
    D. croup

    Croup

15. Which drug is generally given before bronchography?
    A. penicillin
    B. atropine
    C. Valium
    D. Demerol

    atropine

16. How is Dionosil eliminated from the bronchial tree after bronchography?
    A. absorbed from the lung and excreted via the kidney
    B. absorbed from the lung and excreted via the gastrointestinal tract
    C. coughed up
    D. excreted via the sweat glands

    cough up

17. Which of the following is *not* a satisfactory method to introduce contrast to perform bronchography?
    A. directly into the trachea through the cricothyroid membrane
    B. catheter placement through the nose
    C. catheter placement through the mouth
    D. all of the above are satisfactory

    all of the above are satisfactory

EXERCISE VIII-4

Match each of the following with the correct definition by placing the letter of the answer in the space provided. Each question has only one correct answer.

A. dyspnea

B. pleural effusion

C. chronic bronchitis

D. hydatid disease

E. pneumonitis

F. centrilobular emphysema

G. lobar pneumonia

H. pneumothorax

I. hyaline membrane disease

J. compensating emphysema

K. *Pneumocystis carinii*

L. aspiration pneumonia

M. nodular metastatic carcinoma

N. bronchiectasis

O. tuberculosis

P. abscess

Q. hemothorax

R. bronchogenic carcinoma

S. asthma

T. atelectasis

U. empyema

V. apnea

W. pulmonary edema

X. pleurisy

Y. adult respiratory distress syndrome

Z. pneumonic metastatic carcinoma

asthma   1. __S__ caused by infection or allergies which cause mucosal swelling
asthma

bronchogenic carci.2. __R__ chest films show a rounded opacity; currently the leading tumor in men
bronchogenic carcinoma

atelectasis   3. __T__ the condition of a collapsed lung
atelectasis

Chronic bronchitis 4. __C__ most commonly associated with emphysema
chronic bronchitis

bronchiectasis   5. __N__ dilation of smaller bronchi of the lung
bronchiectasis

empyema   6. __U__ pus in the pleural cavity
empyema

abscess   7. __P__ chest radiograph shows air fluid levels with a cavity; a thick wall surrounds the cavity
abscess

hydatid diease

8. __D__ cysts in the lung *hydatid diease*

pleuracy

9. __X__ condition of having inflammation of the pleura

pleurcy

hemothorax

10. __Q__ blood in the pleural cavity

lobar pneumonia

11. __G__ affected lobe shows as a radiopaque area on the chest radiograph

pleural effusion

12. __B__ fluid in the pleural cavity

pleural effusion

pneumothorax

13. __H__ air in the pleural cavity

pneumothorax

hyaline membrane diease

14. __I__ caused by a deficiency of surfactant called lipoprotein in the alveoli of the lung of a premature infant

hyaline membrane diease

tuberculosis

15. __O__ radiograph demonstrates cavitation and calcification

tuberculosis

pneumonitis

16. __E__ inflammation of the lungs

pneumonitis

dyspnea

17. __A__ shortness of breath

dyspnea

nodular metastatic carcinoma

18. __M__ lung carcinoma that appears as multiple round masses throughout the lungs

nodular metastatic carcinoma

abscess

19. __P__ localized necrosis of tissues surrounded by inflammatory debris

abscess

pleurisy

20. __W__ fluid in the lungs

pleurisy

CHAPTER VIII SELF-TEST

There are 50 possible points on this self-test. Score it against the answers found in the exercises. A score of 47 points or higher indicates mastery and retention of this material.

Complete the blanks in the following statements.

1. What radiographic procedure is often required to confirm the diagnosis of bronchiectasis when routine chest radiographs are inconclusive? __bronchography__

2. Obstruction of a bronchus is the most common cause

of ___*atelectasis*___ .

3. What is the name of the area of bifurcation of the

trachea? ___*Couna*___

4. The functional unit for gas exchange in the lungs is

the ___*alveoli*___ .

5. Permanent dilation of the bronchi is known

as ___*bronchiectasis*___ .

6. When a characteristic inverted wedge-shaped opacity of the lung is seen on a radiograph, it may indicate the presence of

a ___*pulmonary embolism*___ .

7. Name the two categories of iodinated contrast media used in bronchograms.

___*aqueous*___   ___*oily*___

8. When areas of fluid consolidation collapse and oppose each other, they cause the bronchi to become visible. This is known as what radiographic

sign? ___*air bronchogram*___

9. Name the layers of the pleura of the lung.

___*viceral*___   ___*parietal*___

10. Which hilum should always appear higher on the

radiograph? ___*left lingua*___

11. The confluence of major bronchi and vessels in each lung is called

the _hilum_____ .

12. Name the four divisions of the mediastinum that are used when defining pathology.

_anterior_____   _superior_____

_posterior_____   _middle_____

13. Supine chest films are unacceptable because they cause the appearance of what

pathology of the heart? _Congestive heart failure_

14. In the lung, a localized necrosis of tissue is known as an

_____abscess_____ .

Mark the following statements "T" for true or "F" for false.

F _____ 15. Rotation of the patient during chest radiography may cause the appearance of ~~loss of lung volume~~. Congestive heart failure

F _____ 16. ~~Pneumonia~~ is a term used to describe an inflammation of the bronchus. Bronchitis

F _____ 17. When a pneumothorax is suspected, the radiographer should take ~~double~~ single exposure inhalation-exhalation films of the chest.

T _____ 18. Leather lung disease is so called because the lung becomes stiff and brittle.

T _____ 19. One common reason for obtaining a chest radiograph is a patient history of asthma.

F _____ 20. Heart magnification is greater on a P~~A~~ AP chest radiograph than it is on an ~~AP~~ PA radiograph.

T _____ 21. Calcification in a coin lesion of the lung usually means the lesion is benign.

T _____ 22. Pleurisy refers to an inflammation of the lining of the lungs.

T   23. Lobar pneumonia mostly involves lung alveoli of an entire lobe.

bronchi

F   24. Bronchitis is the medical term for infection of the ~~air sacs~~ within the lungs.

Circle the letter in front of the correct answer.

25. Which of the following is *not* part of the mediastinum?
    A. heart
    B. lungs
    C. trachea
    D. lymph tissue

26. How is Dionosil eliminated from the bronchial tree after bronchography?
    A. absorbed from the lung and excreted via the kidney
    B. absorbed from the lung and excreted via the gastrointestinal tract
    C. coughed up
    D. excreted via the sweat glands

27. An overexpanded lung can cause all of the following *except*
    A. mediastinal shift
    B. atelectasis
    C. flattened hemidiaphragm
    D. pleural effusion

28. Which of the following is responsible for air exchange?
    A. diaphragm
    B. hilus
    C. alveolus
    D. bronchus

29. Which of the following structures can be well demonstrated on a lateral chest projection?
    A. trachea
    B. interlobar fissure
    C. bronchi
    D. mediastinum

30. Which portion of the mediastinum is *not* used in radiography?
    A. superior
    B. anterior
    C. middle
    D. posterior

31. If an upright chest radiograph cannot be performed, what position is used to demonstrate pleural effusion?
    A. cross table lateral
    B. transthoracic
    C. lateral decubitus
    D. Trendelenburg

32. What is the most common change seen on a routine, yearly chest radiograph?
    A. increased heart size
    B. emphysema
    C. pleurisy
    D. pericardial effusion

33. Patient rotation can be evaluated on a PA chest radiograph by assessing
    A. the curvature of the thoracic spine
    B. the scapula in the lung fields
    C. sternoclavicular joint asymmetry
    D. the height of the clavicles

34. To check for deep inspiration in an adult, the diaphragm should be at which level?
    A. T-11
    B. T-8
    C. T-12
    D. sternal notch

35. Which drug is generally given before bronchography?
    A. penicillin
    B. atropine
    C. Valium
    D. Demerol

36. Which of the following chest pathologies would require a decrease in technique from a "normal" chest radiograph?
    A. atelectasis
    B. pneumothorax
    C. pleural effusion
    D. pneumonia

37. The carina is found at the level of
    A. C-7
    B. T-2
    C. T-5
    D. T-8

38. Anterior oblique views of the chest demonstrate all but the
    A. heart
    B. aortic arch
    C. pulmonary artery
    D. abdominal aorta

Match each of the following with the correct definition by placing the letter of the correct answer in the space provided. Each question has only one correct answer.

A. dyspnea

B. pleural effusion

C. chronic bronchitis

D. hydatid disease

E. pneumonitis

F. centrilobular emphysema

G. lobar pneumonia

H. pneumothorax

I. hyaline membrane disease

J. compensating emphysema

K. *Pneumocystis carinii*

L. aspiration pneumonia

M. nodular metastatic carcinoma

N. bronchiectasis

Q. tuberculosis

P. abscess

Q. hemothorax

R. bronchogenic carcinoma

S. asthma

T. atelectasis

U. empyema

V. apnea

W. pulmonary edema

X. pleurisy

Y. adult respiratory distress syndrome

Z. pneumonic metastatic carcinoma

39. __T__ the condition of a collapsed lung

40. __B__ fluid in the lungs

41. __G__ affected lobe shows as a radiopaque area on the chest radiograph

42. __R__ chest films show a rounded opacity; currently the leading tumor in men

43. __H__ air in the pleural cavity

44. __X__ condition of having inflammation of the pleura

45. __O__ radiograph demonstrates cavitation and calcification

46. __M__ lung carcinoma that appears as multiple round masses throughout the lungs

47. __P__ chest radiograph shows air fluid levels with a cavity; a thick wall surrounds the cavity

48. __A__ shortness of breath

49. __B__ fluid in the pleural cavity

50. __E__ inflammation of the lungs

Circulatory System

Rationale

As important as the lungs are in a chest radiograph, the size and shape of the heart are equally important. Abnormalities of the heart can be determined during a routine chest radiograph. The aortic arch is easily seen and can be a clue to pathologic conditions to the alert radiographer. Just as in radiography of the lungs, the patient must be properly positioned to determine any pathologic conditions.

The introduction of contrast media into the circulatory system allows the visualization of arterial and venous structures. Radiographers who have specialized in angiography or heart catheterization must be aware of the many changes in the body that indicate potential problems during the examination. Manifestations of arterial insufficiency include changes in skin color and temperature. Ulcerations and gangrene are other manifestations of which the radiographer should be aware that point to circulatory problems.

Examinations of the lymph system require the patient to lie on the x-ray table for long periods of time between radiographs. Not only could the patient experience problems from the procedure, but also the radiographer should be a source of comfort to help pass the time during the examination.

Objectives

1. ( ) Identify the chambers, valves, and major vessels of the heart from a drawing.

2. ( ) Name and describe each of the three types of circulation.

3. ( ) Describe a cardiac series.

4. ( ) Explain the purpose of lymphography.

5. ( ) Define each of the following terms:

( ) atherosclerosis	( ) arteriosclerosis
( ) stenosis	( ) thrombus
( ) cardiomegaly	( ) myocardial infarction
( ) dyspnea	( ) dextrocardia
( ) valvular disease	( ) incompetency
( ) insufficiency	( ) lymphostasis
( ) lymphedema	( ) lymphangitis
( ) lymphadenitis	( ) lymphedema

6. ( ) Name three left-to-right shunts.

7. ( ) Describe tetralogy of Fallot and its manifestations.

8. ( ) List three types of aneurysms.

9. ( ) Explain the difference between left-sided and right-sided heart failure.

10. ( ) Define pericardial effusion.

11. ( )   Describe rheumatic heart disease and its manifestations.

12. ( )   List two types of neoplasms of the lymph system defined in the text.

EXERCISE IX-1

Complete the blanks in the following statements.

1. Identify the anatomic parts indicated.

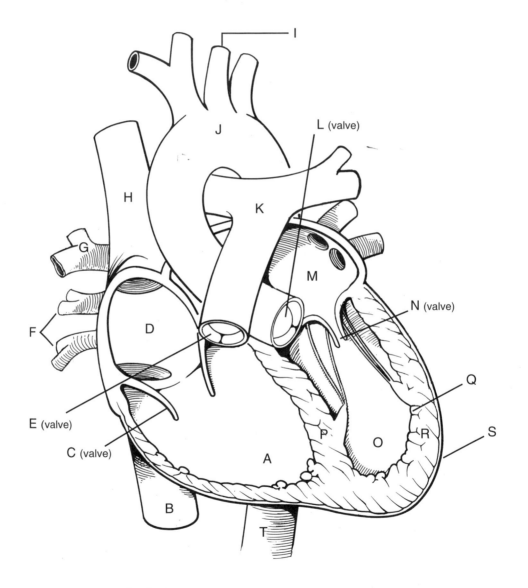

A. r. ventricle   D. r. atrium

B. IVC   E. pulmonary semilunar valve

C. tricuspid valve   F. r. pulmonary veins

G. r. pulmonary artery   N. mitral valve

H. SVC   O. l. ventricle

I. l. common carotid   P. septum

J. aortic arch   Q. endocardium

K. pulmonary artery   R. myocardium

L. aortic semilunar valve S. pericardium

M. l. atrium   T. thoracic aorta

2. Lymph vessels are called _lymphatics_ .

3. Name the two types of lymphatics.

___Superficial___   ___deep___

4. Name three types of aneurysms.

___Saccular___   ___fusiform___

___dissecting___

5. Trace the path of the blood beginning with its return to the heart by the superior vena cava (SVC) and inferior vena cava (IVC). IVC and SVC into the

A. __right atrium__ of the heart, through the

B. __tricuspid valve__ into the

C. __right ventricle__ of the heart. From here it flows through the

(semilunar valve)

D. __pulmonary valve__ into the

E. __pulmonary artery__ , which takes the blood to the

F. _lungs_ _____ to pick up oxygen. Blood returns by way of the

G. _pulmonary vein_ _____ into the

H. _left atrium_ _____ of the heart, through the

I. _mitral valve (bicuspid)_ ___ and into the

J. _left ventricle_ _____ of the heart, which sends oxygenated blood through the

K. _aortic valve_ _____ into the

L. _aorta_ _____ which carries the blood to the body.

6. Name the procedure that uses a balloon to dilate a narrowed coronary artery.

percutaneous transluminal angioplasty

7. Which procedure is best to demonstrate mitral valve stenosis?

ultrasound/echocardiography

8. Name the two causes of pericardial effusion.

tuberculosis   _viral infection_

9. Besides the spleen, what are three other lymph organs?

thymus   _adenoids_

tonsils

EXERCISE IX-2

Mark the following statements "T" for true or "F" for false. If the statement is false, reword it to make it true by changing the incorrect portions.

_F_   1. The term thrombus refers to a ~~tumor found in the heart~~. _blood clot in any vessel_

T ___ (2.) Mitral valve stenosis is the most common heart abnormality associated with rheumatic heart disease.

aquired diesed area

F ___ 3. A myocardial infarction is a ~~form of congenital heart disease.~~
of the heart wall

T ___ 4. The pericardium is the sac enveloping the external surface of the heart.

T ___ 5. Arteriosclerosis is a process of hardening of the arteries.

T ___ 6. The term myocarditis describes an inflammation of the heart muscle.

F ___ 7. Systemic circulation is when (oxygenated) blood goes to the body.

T ___ 8. Pulmonary veins take oxygenated blood to the left atrium.

RAO

F ___ 9. On a cardiac series, the ~~RAO~~ is done at 45 degrees.

LAO – 60°
left

F ___ 10. The ~~right~~ common carotid artery is a branch of the aortic arch.
Right branches off of brachiocephalic

T ___ 11. The contracting phase of the heart is called systole.

left

F ___ 12. The ~~right~~ atrioventricular valve is also called the bicuspid valve.
right atroventricular – tricuspid
left

F ___ 13. Mitral insufficiency allows blood to flow back into the ~~right~~ atrium.

T ___ 14. Lymphangiography is used to assess Hodgkin disease.

T ___ 15. Delayed films in an examination of the lymph system are called lymphadenograms.

NODES

F ___ 16. Lymph ~~ducts~~ are the "filtering" portion of the lymph system.

T ___ 17. Unexplained peripheral swelling is one reason for performing lymphangiography.

T ___ 18. Lymph is continuously being produced from tissue fluid by filtration.

Left

F ___ 19. Contraction of the ~~right~~ ventricle forces oxygenated blood into the aorta.

T ___ 20. Congestive heart failure refers to the inability of the heart to propel sufficient blood to the body.

EXERCISE IX-3

Circle the letter in front of the correct answer.

1. An absolute contraindication for lymphangiography is
   A. thyroid disease because contrast agents contain iodine
   B. known lymphoma
   C. known metastases to the lymph nodes
   D. none of the above

2. To demonstrate lymph channels during lymphography, one would obtain radiographs
   A. during injection and up to 6 hours postinjection
   B. 6–24 hours postinjection
   C. 24–72 hours postinjection
   D. 3–7 days postinjection

   during injection and up t 6hrs posting.

3. All of the following are part of the lymphatic system *except* the
   A. spleen
   B. cisterna chyli
   C. tonsils
   D. pancreas

   drains from lower extremity

   pancreas

4. How much contrast material is usually needed to visualize adequately the lymphatics of the lower extremity and the lymph nodes when performing lymphography by injection into the foot?
   A. 2 mL
   B. 4 mL
   C. 8 mL
   D. 50 mL

   8mls

5. When performing lymphadenography, how long after the injection is the examination made?
   A. 1 hour
   B. 3 hours
   C. 12 hours
   D. 24 hours

   24hrs

6. The amount of contrast media used in lymphangiography over a 30-minute period is
   A. 1 mL
   B. 4 mL
   C. 6 mL
   D. 10 mL

   6mls   30~6

7. What is *not* true regarding lymphangiography?
   A. The examination can take up to several hours just to inject the contrast material.
   B. The patient may need stitches to close the incision.
   C. The technologist can inject the contrast material quickly.
   D. Both lower extremities can be performed at the same time.

8. When lymphangiography is performed, a blue dye is usually injected
   A. into the saphenous vein
   B. between the first and second toe
   C. between the ankle and the knee
   D. into the superior lateral region of the foot

9. Which is *not* a lymphatic duct?
   A. cisterna magnum duct
   B. cisterna chyli duct
   C. thoracic duct
   D. left duct

10. How is contrast material introduced in a lymphangiogram?
    A. ingestion
    B. direct injection
    C. indirect injection
    D. buccal

11. Which duct narrows to form the thoracic duct?
    A. cisterna chyli
    B. cisterna magna
    C. right thoracic duct
    D. left lymphatic duct

12. In lymphangiography, the contrast agent usually used is
    A. Evans blue
    B. Renografin
    C. Ethiodol
    D. direct sky blue

13. The smallest of all blood vessels are called
    A. arteries
    B. capillaries
    C. venules
    D. arterioles

14. Which of the following is *not* a major cause of pericardial effusion?
    A. myocardial infarct
    B. tuberculosis
    C. mycobacteria
    D. infection

15. Which is *not* a branch off the aortic arch?
    A. brachiocephalic
    B. innominate
    C. left subclavian
    D. right common carotid

16. Air in the mediastinum is known as
    A. pleural effusion
    B. hemothorax
    C. pneumothorax
    D. pneumomediastinum

17. Poor inspiration on a chest radiograph causes the appearance of what pathology?
    A. COPD
    B. CVA
    C. CHF
    D. MI

18. Which of the following does *not* make up the pulmonary window?
    A. pulmonary great vessels
    B. carina
    C. cupula
    D. left main stem bronchus

19. The degenerative disease in which the walls of the arteries lose elasticity from hardening is known as
    A. arteriosclerosis
    B. arterionecrosis
    C. athetosis
    D. arteriostenosis

20. Blood is transported via the four pulmonary veins to the
    A. left ventricle
    B. aorta
    C. superior vena cava
    D. left atrium

21. At about the level of L-4, the abdominal aorta bifurcates into the
    A. left and right common iliac arteries
    B. right and left femoral arteries
    C. left and right common carotid arteries
    D. right and left celiac arteries

22. The mitral valve of the heart is correctly described as
    (1) located between the left atrium and ventricle (2) having three cusps
    (3) open during ventricular diastole
    A. 1 and 2
    B. 2 and 3
    C. 1 and 3
    D. 1, 2, and 3

23. A stationary blood clot that has formed within a blood vessel is known as a(n)
    A. embolus
    B. hematoma
    C. thrombus
    D. hemangioma

24. What radiographic method is used for examining the chambers of the heart?
    A. angiocardiography
    B. selective coronary arteriography
    C. peripheral angiography
    D. celiac arteriography

25. Which of the following occur(s) during ventricular diastole?
    (1) the semilunar valves remain closed   (2) the ventricles of the heart fill with blood   (3) the atrioventricular valves open
    A.   1 only
    B.   2 only
    C.   3 only
    D.   1, 2, and 3

26. The circulation that takes blood to the body is the
    A.   pulmonary circulation
    B.   systemic circulation
    C.   portal circulation
    D.   cardiac circulation

27. What vessels send oxygenated blood to the heart muscle?
    A.   right and left coronary veins
    B.   right and left coronary arteries
    C.   right coronary artery and left coronary vein
    D.   right coronary vein and left coronary artery

28. The coeur en sabot appearance is associated with
    A.   right ventricle enlargement
    B.   asthma
    C.   cardiomegaly
    D.   patent ductus arteriosus

29. The type of aneurysm that usually begins as a tear in the layers of the artery wall is
    A.   stenosis
    B.   fusiform
    C.   saccular
    D.   dissecting

30. The most common cause of congestive heart failure in the older adult is
    A.   hypertensive heart disease
    B.   low blood pressure
    C.   cor pulmonale
    D.   coarctation of the aorta

EXERCISE IX-4

Match each of the following with the correct definition by placing the letter of the answer in the space provided. Each question has only one correct answer.

A. arteriosclerotic heart disease

B. congestive heart disease

C. lymphadenitis

D. dissecting aneurysm

E. tetralogy of Fallot

F. lymphostasis

G. rheumatic heart disease

H. rib notching

I. pericardial effusion

J. hypertensive heart disease

K. septal defects

L. lymphangitis

M. pericarditis

N. thrombus

O. endocarditis

P. stenosis

Q. lymphedema

R. dextrocardia *situs inversus*

S. arteriosclerosis

T. coarctation of the aorta

U. ectasia

1. __N__ blood clot found inside a vessel or the heart

    thrombus

2. __M__ inflammation of the pericardium

    pericarditis

3. __P__ narrowing of the lumen of a vessel

    stenosis

4. __R__ when the heart is located on the right side of the body

    dextracardia

5. __S__ hardening of the arteries

    arteriosclerosis

6. __K__ small openings in the septum of the heart that are congenital

    septal defects

7. __O__ inflammation of the heart valves

    endocarditis

8. __E__ most common cause of blue baby

    tetralogy of fallot

9. __I__ fluid in the pericardial sac

    pericardeal effusion

10. __D__ hemorrhage that occurs between the layers of the wall of the artery

    dissecting aneurysm

11. __U__ uniform dilation of the entire portion of the distal aorta

    ectasia

12. __A__ caused by plaque buildup in the coronary arteries and can cause a myocardial infarct

    arteriosclerotic heart disease

13. __B__ chest radiograph shows a pulmonary vascular shift and increased heart size; usually occurs in elderly individuals whose hearts must pump against the increased pressure owing to hypertension

    congestive heart failure

14. __G__ calcification of the mitral valve as seen on a chest x-ray is the indication of this

    rheumatic heart disease

15. __H__ caused by anastomotic vessels enlarging from increased volume and causing pressure erosions on the ribs

    rib notching

16. __I__ cause of enlargement of the left ventricle and rib notching

    coarctation of the aorta

17. __F__ obstruction and dilation of the lymph system

    lymphostasis

18. __L__ inflammation of lymphatic channels   *c/o*

    lymphangitis

19. __C__ inflammation of lymph nodes   *n/d*

    lymphadenitis

20. __Q__ hypoplasia and maldevelopment of the lymph system

    lymphedema

A. fluoroscopy

B. cardiac series

C. ultrasonography

D. aortography

E. cardiography

F. nuclear medicine

Coumadin 1, 2, 2½, 3. 4, 5 7, 10, is a blood thinner

December 10 Chapter 10-11

common place for plaque build up is Carotids   Siphon also

thin membrane   berry anurism
                     circle of willis

21. _A_ study done to localize calcifications in the chest or heart

22. _F_ known as a gated heart scan

23. _B_ a four-view chest examination that shows the pulmonary window

24. _E_ examination of the chambers of the heart with contrast media

25. _D_ study of the abdominal aorta

_B_

cardiac series

26. _A_ uses barium to outline the esophagus to show its reference to the chambers of the heart

27. _C_ examination that is best to evaluate septal defects

28. _C_ echocardiography

29. _F_ radionuclide thallium perfusion scan

30. _A_ by itself, it is limited in value; best used in cardiac series

---

CHAPTER IX SELF-TEST

There are 50 possible points on this self-test. Score it against the answers found in the exercises. A score of 47 points or higher indicates mastery and retention of this material.

Complete the blanks in the following statements.

1. Which procedure is best to demonstrate mitral valve stenosis?

   ultrasound / echocardiography

2. Name three types of aneurysms.

   fusiform   _sacular_

   dissecting

   in coronaries — lesions/
   occlusions — where plaque builds up

3. Besides the spleen, what are three other lymph organs?

thymus _adenoids_

tonsils

4. Name the procedure that uses a balloon to dilate a narrowed coronary artery.

percutaneous transluminal angioplasty

5. Lymph vessels are called _lymphatics_ .

6. Name the two causes of pericardial effusion.

tuberculosis _viral infection_

Mark the following statements "T" for true or "F" for false.

_T_ 7. Congestive heart failure refers to the inability of the heart to propel sufficient blood to the body.

_T_ 8. Lymphangiography is used to assess Hodgkin disease.

_F_ 9. On a cardiac series, the ~~LAO~~ RAO is done at 45 degrees.

_T_ 10. Arteriosclerosis is a process of hardening of the arteries. LAD 60

_F_ 11. Lymph ~~ducts~~ NODES are the "filtering" portion of the lymph system.

_T_ 12. Mitral valve stenosis is the most common heart abnormality associated with rheumatic heart disease.

_T_ 13. Delayed films in an examination of the lymph system are called lymphadenograms.

_F_ 14. The ~~right~~ left common carotid artery is a branch of the aortic arch.

Circle the letter in front of the correct answer.

15. What is *not* true regarding lymphangiography?
    A. The examination can take up to several hours just to inject the contrast material.
    B. The patient may need stitches to close the incision.
    C. The technologist can inject the contrast material quickly.
    D. Both lower extremities can be performed at the same time.

16. To demonstrate lymph channels during lymphography, one would obtain radiographs
    A. during injection and up to 6 hours postinjection
    B. 6–24 hours postinjection
    C. 24–72 hours postinjection
    D. 3–7 days postinjection

17. How much contrast material is usually needed to visualize adequately the lymphatics of the lower extremity and the lymph nodes when performing lymphography by injection into the foot?
    A. 2 mL
    B. 4 mL
    C. 8 mL
    D. 50 mL

18. Which of the following is *not* a major cause of pericardial effusion?
    A. myocardial infarct
    B. tuberculosis
    C. mycobacteria
    D. infection

19. When lymphangiography is performed, a blue dye is usually injected
    A. into the saphenous vein
    B. between the first and second toe
    C. between the ankle and the knee
    D. into the superior lateral region of the foot

20. An absolute contraindication for lymphangiography is
    A. thyroid disease because contrast agents contain iodine
    B. known lymphoma
    C. known metastases to the lymph nodes
    D. none of the above

21. In lymphangiography, the contrast agent usually used is
    A. Evans blue
    B. Renografin
    C. Ethiodol
    D. direct sky blue

22. The type of aneurysm that usually begins as a tear in the layers of the artery wall is
    A. stenosis
    B. fusiform
    C. saccular
    D. dissecting

23. The amount of contrast media used in lymphangiography over a 30-minute period is
    A. 1 mL
    B. 4 mL
    C. 6 mL
    D. 10 mL

24. Poor inspiration on a chest radiograph causes the appearance of what pathology?
    A. COPD
    B. CVA
    C. CHF
    D. MI

25. Which of the following occur(s) during ventricular diastole?
    (1) The semilunar valves remain closed   (2) The ventricles of the heart fill with blood   (3) The atrioventricular valves open
    A. 1 only
    B. 2 only
    C. 3 only
    D. 1, 2, and 3

26. The mitral valve of the heart is correctly described as
    (1) located between the left atrium and ventricle   (2) having three cusps (3) open during ventricular diastole
    A. 1 and 2
    B. 2 and 3
    C. 1 and 3
    D. 1, 2, and 3

27. When performing lymphadenography, how long after the injection is the examination made?
    A. 1 hour
    B. 3 hours
    C. 12 hours
    D. 24 hours

28. Which of the following does *not* make up the pulmonary window?
    A. pulmonary great vessels
    B. carina
    C. cupula
    D. left main stem bronchus

29. What radiographic method is used for examining the chambers of the heart?
    A. angiocardiography
    B. selective coronary arteriography
    C. peripheral angiography
    D. celiac arteriography

30. The most common cause of congestive heart failure in the older adult is
    A. hypertensive heart disease
    B. low blood pressure
    C. cor pulmonale
    D. coarctation of the aorta

31. Air in the mediastinum is known as
    A. pleural effusion
    B. hemothorax
    C. pneumothorax
    D. pneumomediastinum

32. The coeur en sabot appearance is associated with
    A. right ventricle enlargement
    B. asthma
    C. cardiomegaly
    D. patent ductus arteriosus

33. The degenerative disease in which the walls of the arteries lose elasticity from hardening is known as
    A. arteriosclerosis
    B. arterionecrosis
    C. athetosis
    D. arteriostenosis

Match each of the following with the correct definition by placing the letter of the answer in the space provided. Each question has only one correct answer.

A. arteriosclerotic heart disease   L. lymphangitis

B. congestive heart disease   M. pericarditis

C. lymphadenitis   N. thrombus

D. dissecting aneurysm   O. endocarditis

E. tetralogy of Fallot   P. stenosis

F. lymphostasis   Q. lymphedema

G. rheumatic heart disease   R. dextrocardia

H. rib notching   S. arteriosclerosis

 I. pericardial effusion   T. coarctation of the aorta

J. hypertensive heart disease   U. ectasia

K. septal defects

34. H (T) caused by anastomotic vessels enlarging from increased volume and causing pressure erosions on the ribs

35. C inflammation of lymph nodes

36. M inflammation of the pericardium

37. I fluid in the pericardial sac

38. B chest radiograph shows a pulmonary vascular shift and increased heart size; usually occurs in elderly individuals whose hearts must pump against the increased pressure owing to hypertension

39. R when the heart is located on the right side of the body

40. E most common cause of blue baby

41. Q, F obstruction and dilation of the lymph system

42. K small openings in the septum of the heart that are congenital

43. T cause of enlargement of the left ventricle and rib notching

44. G calcification of the mitral valve as seen on a chest x-ray is the indication of this

- Multiple Choice
- T/F
- Matching

A. fluoroscopy

B. cardiac series

C. ultrasonography

D. aortography

E. cardiography

F. nuclear medicine

45. _A_ study done to localize calcifications in the chest or heart

46. _A_ by itself, it is limited in value; best used in cardiac series

47. _B_ a four-view chest examination that shows the pulmonary window

48. _C_ examination that is best to evaluate septal defects.

49. _E_ examination of the chambers of the heart with contrast media

50. _D_ uses barium to outline the esophagus to show its reference to the chambers of the heart

Nervous System

Rationale

The radiographer is responsible for producing quality films of the skull that allow the radiologist to make a proper diagnosis. Underpenetrated or overpenetrated skull films may obscure a slight density change in the bone, which would otherwise indicate a mass within the brain tissue. Likewise, erosion of the sella can be easily missed if the radiographer does not take the time to make sure the patient is not rotated or tilted. In addition to the patient position, the radiographic tube must be angled properly to project overlying anatomy away from areas that must be demonstrated clearly.

Many of the patients that come to the radiography department have been severely injured, and the technologist must be alert to outward signs of trauma to the head that may not be clearly seen on the radiograph. Ingenuity and creative positioning of patients that are unable to be moved around are often necessary to provide the radiographs required to demonstrate a fracture.

Objectives

1. ( ) Identify the ventricles and related foramina from drawings.

2. ( ) List the three meninges in order from innermost to outermost.

3. ( ) Name the components of the peripheral and automatic nervous systems.

4. ( ) Name the four functions of the cerebrum.

5. ( ) List the functions of the medulla oblongata.

6. ( ) Describe discography.

7. ( ) Explain the difference between lumbar and cervical punctures in myelography.

8. ( ) Define anencephaly and microcephaly.

9. ( ) List the three types of hydrocephaly and describe them.

10. ( ) Name three defects associated with spina bifida.

11. ( ) List the three types of meningitis.

12. ( ) Describe how encephalitis affects the brain.

13. ( ) Explain the difference between concussion and contusion.

14. ( ) Name three types of gliomas.

15. ( ) Define two types of pineal tumors.

16. ( ) Name three types of spinal cord disease discussed in the text.

EXERCISE X-1

1. Identify the anatomic parts indicated.

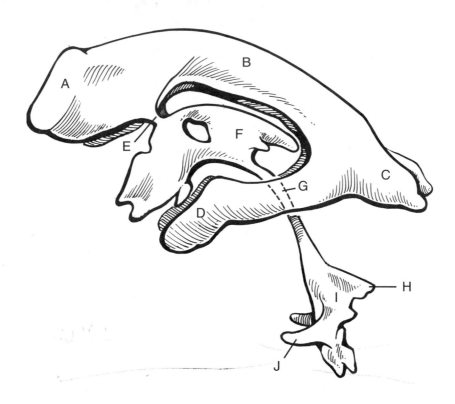

A. _anterior horn_

B. _Body of lateral ventricle_

C. _posterior horn_

D. _inferior horn_

E. _foramen of Monro_

F. _3rd ventricle_

G. _aqueduct of Sylvius_

H. _posterior superior recess_

I. _4th ventricle_

J. _foramen of luschka_

Complete the blanks in the following statements.

2. The pathologic condition that refers to dilation of the ventricular system is called *hydrocephalis* .

3. When lumbar punctures are not possible, where is the puncture made for a subarachnoid myelogram? *Cervical area - cistera magna*

4. The heart rate is controlled by which nervous system?

autonomic system

5. List the three systems that make up the nervous system.

Central   *peripheral*

autonomic

6. What is another name for the central nervous system?

Cerebrospinal system

7. What are the two main components of the central nervous system?

brain   *spinal cord*

8. The cells of the nervous system are called

neurons .

9. List the three divisions of the brain.

cerebrum
cerebellum ⟶ *forebrain*

midbrain   *hindbrain*

mesocephalon ↓   *itself* ✗

10. What structures are found in the diencephalon?

thalmus   3rd ventricle

hypothalmus

P 241

11. Name a function of the midbrain. auditory reflexes

12. What is formed in the ventricles of the brain?

Cerebrospinal fluid

13. Name the three meninges in order from innermost to outermost.

pia mater   dura mater

arachnoid

14. What are the leptomeninges? pia & arachnoid meniges

15. Name the two divisions of the autonomic nervous system.

sympathic   parasympatic

16. What two contrast agents are used in negative contrast myelograms?

air   oxygen

17. What happens to the patient's brain if pressure from hydrocephalus is not

relieved? brain may herniate toward the
foramen magnum

18. What are the two types of shunts used in treatment of hydrocephalus?

ventriculoatrial   ventriculoperitioneal

19. A common malformation in which the posterior arches and spinous processes of some vertebrae fail to close or are absent is known as

spina bifida .

20. When the malformation of the vertebrae is limited to the <u>neural arch,</u> the condition is called _spina bifida oculta_ .

21. List the three conditions that may coexist with a spina bifida.

meningocele   _myelomeningocele_

myelocele

22. What are two causes of aneurysms in middle-aged patients?

atheroma   _hypertension_

23. Where do most cerebral aneurysms occur?

circle of Willis

24. Sixty percent of all strokes are due to _emboli_ .

25. Name the four types of hematomas.

subdural   _subarachnoid_

epidural   _intracerebral_

26. What are three common types of skull fractures?

linear   _comminuted_

depressed

27. Name the four common head injuries.

concussion   *fracture*

contusion   *hemorrhage*

28. A complication of an empyema is _*osteomylitis*_ .

29. Benign gliomas are called _*astrocytomas*_ .

30. Which two intracranial tumors can affect sight?

pituitary adenoma   *craniopharyngioma*

31. What is the hallmark sign of neurofibromas?

foraminal widening

32. Blood and cerebrospinal fluid mix to create this sign, which is indicative of a basilar skull fracture. The sign is called

halo sign .

EXERCISE X-2

Mark the following statements "T" for true or "F" for false. If it is a false statement, reword it to make it true by changing the incorrect portions.

_*T*_ 1. The most common brain hemorrhage is the subdural.

_*T*_ 2. The ventricular system of the brain consists of four ventricles.

_*T*_ 3. Epidural myelography has a puncture site at the sacral hiatus.

_*T*_ 4. The epidural space is between the dura mater and the vertebral canal.

_*F*_ 5. The most common primary brain tumor is a ~~meningioma~~. *glioma*

_*F*_ 6. Most myelograms ~~are epidural myelograms~~. *subarachnoid* *sub arachnoid*

_T_   7. If the patient presents with tumors or herniated discs, an epidural myelogram is performed.

_T_   8. Three major causes of stroke are thrombus, embolism, and hemorrhage.

_F_   9. Spina bifida with meningeal protrusion is referred to as ~~myelocele~~. *meningiocle*

_T_   10. CT is currently the method of choice for demonstrating spinal cord abscesses and neoplasms.

EXERCISE X-3

Circle the letter in front of the correct answer.

1. Which of the following contains cerebrospinal fluid?
   A. subarachnoid
   B. pia mater
   C. dura mater
   D. extradural space

2. Trace the path of the cerebrospinal fluid.
   A. lateral ventricles—aqueduct of Sylvius—third ventricle—fourth ventricle—foramina of Luschka and Magendie—subarachnoid space
   B. aqueduct of Sylvius—lateral ventricles—foramina of Luschka and Magendie—third ventricle—fourth ventricle—subarachnoid space
   C. lateral ventricles—foramen of Monro—third ventricle—aqueduct of Sylvius—fourth ventricle—foramina of Luschka and Magendie—subarachnoid space
   D. foramina of Luschka and Magendie—lateral ventricles—interventricular foramen—third ventricle—aqueduct of Sylvius—fourth ventricle—subarachnoid space

3. Methods of injecting contrast media for myelography are all of the following *except*
   A. lumbar puncture
   B. cisternal puncture
   C. sacral hiatus puncture
   D. thoracic puncture

4. Which of the following is *not* a membrane covering the brain?
   A. dura mater
   B. pia mater
   C. arachnoid
   D. epidura

5. In performing a routine myelogram, the contrast material is injected into which space?
   A. epidural space
   B. subdural space
   C. subarachnoid space
   D. cisterna magna

6. The anterior and inferior horns are part of which of the following?
   A. lateral ventricles
   B. third ventricle
   C. fourth ventricle
   D. foramina of Magendie and Luschka

7. The third and fourth ventricles are connected by the
   A. aqueduct of Sylvius
   B. foramen of Monro
   C. foramen of Magendie
   D. foramen of Luschka

8. In the adult, the spinal cord ends
   A. in the coccyx
   B. in the sacrum
   C. at L4-L5
   D. at L1-L2

9. How many ventricles are present in the brain?
   A. 2
   B. 3
   C. 4
   D. variable

10. Cerebrospinal fluid circulates primarily in which meningeal space?
   A. subarachnoid
   B. epidural
   C. subdural
   D. subpial

11. During myelography, a protrusion into the spinal canal
   A. gives a smooth, symmetric outline to the column of contrast
   B. is not demonstrated on a cross-table lateral
   C. shows as a defect in the outline of the bolus of contrast material
   D. is demonstrated only on oblique-position radiographs

12. The puncture site for myelography is usually between
   A. T-12 and L-1
   B. L-1 and L-2
   C. L-3 and L-4
   D. L-5 and S-1

13. Which of the following types of contrast media are employed in myelography?
   (1) Negative—gaseous medium   (2) Positive—aqueous iodinated medium
   (3) Positive—oily iodinated medium
   A. 1 and 2
   B. 1 and 3
   C. 2 and 3
   D. 1, 2, and 3

14. Which of the following are true regarding the spinal cord?
    (1) It extends from the medulla oblongata to the level of the second lumbar vertebral body   (2) The cord gives rise to 12 pairs of spinal nerves   (3) The pia mater is a protective membrane in contact with the cord
    A. 1 and 2
    B. 1 and 3
    C. 2 and 3
    D. 1, 2, and 3

15. A hematoma occurring after a blunt head injury to the frontal or occipital area is probably a
    A. subdural hematoma
    B. subarachnoid hematoma
    C. epidural hematoma
    D. intracerebral hematoma

16. What term denotes a rapid shift of the brain within the cranium and striking the adjacent wall resulting in unconsciousness?
    A. contusion
    B. concussion
    C. contracoup
    D. edema

17. Brain metastases have a primary source from what two areas?
    A. bladder, stomach
    B. lung, breast
    C. stomach, breast
    D. breast, cervix

18. A viral inflammation of the meninges is called
    A. meningioma
    B. meningitis
    C. encephalitis
    D. meningocele

EXERCISE X-4

Match each of the following with the correct definition by placing the letter of the answer in the space provided. Each question has only one correct answer.

A. empyema

B. osteomyelitis

C. compensatory hydrocephaly

D. concussion

E. contusion

F. cerebrovascular accident

G. hemorrhage

H. meningocele

I. myelomeningocele

J. myelocele

K. internal hydrocephaly

L. external hydrocephaly

M. encephalitis

N. epidural abscess

O. anencephalus

P. meningitis

Q. microcephaly

R. mesencephalon

S. astrocytoma

T. neurofibroma

1. O severe malformation in which there is absence of the cranial vault
anecephalus

2. M inflammation of the brain,
encephalitis

3. K hydrocephalus in only the ventricles
internal encephaly

4. F impairment of the cerebral circulation
cerebrevascular acadent

5. Q exceedingly small head
microcephaly

6. C also known as external hydrocephalus
Compensatory hydrocephaly

7. J protrusion of the cord through the meninges
myelocele

8. N collection of pus between the skull and the underlying dura mater
epidural abscess

9. F commonly referred to as stroke
cerebrovascular accident

10. P inflammation of the leptomeninges
menigitis

11. G escape of blood from the vessels into the cranial vault
hemorrhage

12. R midbrain
mesencephalen

13. D most common head injury -
concussion

14. B common complication of an empyema
osteomylitis

15. E bruises on the surface of the brain
contusion

16. S benign form of glioma
astrocytoma

17. I meninges and spinal cord herniate through a spinal defect
myelomeningcele

18. H protrusion of the meninges through a spinal defect
meningocele

19. A most commonly caused by spread of infection from the sinuses
empyema

20. I primary spinal neoplasm
neurofibroma

CHAPTER X SELF-TEST

There are 50 possible points on this self-test. Score it against the answers found in the exercises. A score of 47 points or higher indicates mastery and retention of this material.

Complete the blanks in the following statements.

1. List the three systems that make up the nervous system.

   Automatic   *peripheral*

   central

2. What is formed in the ventricles of the brain?

   CSF (Cerebrospinal fluid

3. What are the two main components of the central nervous system?

   brain   *spinal cord*

4. List the three conditions that may coexist with a spina bifida.

   meningocele   *myelocele*

   myelomeningocele

5. What are three common types of skull fractures?

   Comminuted   *depressed*

   linear

6. What happens to the patient's brain if pressure from hydrocephalus is not relieved? *brain may herniate towards foramen magnum*

7. When lumbar punctures are not possible, where is the puncture made for a subarachnoid myelogram? *cervical area*

cistern magna

8. A common malformation in which the posterior arches and spinous processes of some vertebrae fail to close or are absent is known as

Spina bifida.

9. Name the four types of hematomas.

subdural   *subarachnoid*

epidural   *intracerebral*

10. Blood and cerebrospinal fluid mix to create this sign, which is indicative of a basilar skull fracture. The sign is called

halo sign.

11. The pathologic condition that refers to dilation of the ventricular system is called *hydrocephalus*.

12. Name the four common head injuries.

concussion   *fracture*

contussion   *hemorrhage*

13. Name the three meninges in order from innermost to outermost.

① *pia mater*   ② *arachnoid*

③ *dura mater*

14. What two contrast agents are used in negative contrast myelograms?

air   *negative*

15. Where do most cerebral aneurysms occur?

Circle of Willis

16. What are the leptomeninges? *pia & arachnoid meninges*

17. What is the hallmark sign of neurofibromas?

foraminal widening

18. Sixty percent of all strokes are due to ___ *emboli* .

19. The cells of the nervous system are

called ___ *neurons* .

20. When the malformation of the vertebrae is limited to the neural arch, the

condition is called *spina bifida occulta* .

Mark the following statement "T" for true or "F" for false.

_F_ 21. The most common primary brain tumor is a *subdural* ~~meningioma~~.

_T_ 22. Three major causes of stroke are thrombus, embolism, and hemorrhage.

_T_ 23. The ventricular system of the brain consists of four ventricles.

_T_ 24. CT is currently the method of choice for demonstrating spinal cord abscesses and neoplasms.

_F_ *subarachnoid*

_____ 25. Most myelograms are ~~epidural mye~~lograms.

_T_

_____ 26. The epidural space is between the dura mater and the vertebral canal.

Circle the letter in front of the correct answer.

27. A viral inflammation of the meninges is called
    A. meningioma
    B. meningitis
    C. encephalitis
    D. meningocele

28. In the adult, the spinal cord ends
    A. in the coccyx
    B. in the sacrum
    C. at L4-L5
    D. at L1-L2

29. A hematoma occurring after a blunt head injury to the frontal or occipital area is probably a
    A. subdural hematoma
    B. subarachnoid hematoma
    C. epidural hematoma
    D. intracerebral hematoma

30. Which of the following types of contrast media are employed in myelography?
    (1) Negative—gaseous medium   (2) Positive—aqueous iodinated medium
    (3) Positive—oily iodinated medium
    A. 1 and 2
    B. 1 and 3
    C. 2 and 3
    D. 1, 2, and 3

31. During myelography, a protrusion into the spinal canal
    A. gives a smooth, symmetric outline to the column of contrast
    B. is not demonstrated on a cross-table lateral
    C. shows as a defect in the outline of the bolus of contrast material
    D. is demonstrated only on oblique-position radiographs

32. In performing a routine myelogram, the contrast material is injected into which space?
    A. epidural space
    B. subdural space
    C. subarachnoid space
    D. cisterna magna

33. Which of the following contains cerebrospinal fluid?
    A. subarachnoid
    B. pia mater
    C. dura mater
    D. extradural space

34. The puncture site for myelography is usually between
    A. T-12 and L-1
    B. L-1 and L-2
    C. L-3 and L-4
    D. L-5 and S-1

35. Brain metastases have a primary source from what two areas?
    A. bladder, stomach
    B. lung, breast
    C. stomach, breast
    D. breast, cervix

36. Methods of injecting contrast media for myelography are all of the following *except*
    A. lumbar puncture
    B. cisternal puncture
    C. sacral hiatus puncture
    D. thoracic puncture

37. Cerebrospinal fluid circulates primarily in which meningeal space?
    A. subarachnoid
    B. epidural
    C. subdural
    D. subpia

38. Which of the following are true regarding the spinal cord?
    (1) It extends from the medulla oblongata to the level of the second lumbar vertebral body (2) The cord gives rise to 12 pairs of spinal nerves (3) The pia mater is a protective membrane in contact with the cord
    A. 1 and 2
    B. 1 and 3
    C. 2 and 3
    D. 1, 2, and 3

39. Trace the path of the cerebrospinal fluid.
    A. lateral ventricles—aqueduct of Sylvius—third ventricle—fourth ventricle—foramina of Luschka and Magendie—subarachnoid space
    B. aqueduct of Sylvius—lateral ventricles—foramina of Luschka and Magendie—third ventricle—fourth ventricle—subarachnoid space
    C. lateral ventricles—foramen of Monro—third ventricle—aqueduct of Sylvius—fourth ventricle—foramina of Luschka and Magendie—subarachnoid space
    D. foramina of Luschka and Magendie—lateral ventricles—interventricular foramen—third ventricle—aqueduct of Sylvius—fourth ventricles—subarachnoid space

40. What term denotes a rapid shift of the brain within the cranium and striking the adjacent wall resulting in unconsciousness?
    A. contusion
    B. concussion
    C. contracoup
    D. edema

Match each of the following with the correct definition by placing the letter of the answer in the space provided. Each question has only one correct answer.

A. empyema

B. osteomyelitis

C. compensatory hydrocephaly

D. concussion

E. contusion

F. cerebrovascular accident

G. hemorrhage

H. meningocele

I. myelomeningocele

J. myelocele

K. internal hydrocephaly

L. external hydrocephaly

M. encephalitis

N. epidural abscess

O. anencephalus

P. meningitis

Q. microcephaly

R. mesencephalon

S. astrocytoma

T. neurofibroma

(41.) C benign form of glioma
astrocytoma

42. G escape of blood from the vessels into the cranial vault
hemorrhage

43. Q exceedingly small head
microcephaly

44. A most commonly caused by spread of infection from the sinuses
empyema

45. D most common head injury
concussion

46. J protrusion of the cord through the meninges
myelocele

47. M inflammation of the brain
encephalitis

48. H protrusion of the meninges through a spinal defect
meningocele

49. E. bruises on the surface of the brain
contussion

50. O severe malformation in which there is absence of the cranial vault
anencephalus

Endocrine System

Thursday Morning

Hereditary

1. Down's Syndrome —
2. Turner's Syndrome — Gonadal — Shorten 4th meta carple
   female urinary abnormalities
   No ovolation!
3. Klinefaltu's Syndrome. Male
4. Marfan's Syndrome — Gonadal — Same as above
   testis dont mature
   ↳ Connecting Tissue defect
      Cardiovascular problems
      dissecting aorting anyersms

Nutritional — vitamins formed only by plants

1. Beriberi — def. 2 catergories
   thymine
   pins & needles sensation
   in extremities
2. Pellagra — lack of niacin
   reddins & scalying of skin
3. Scurvy
   give then niacin
4. Vitamin D
5. Vitamin A
6. Vitamin K

Fat Soluable		Water Soluable	
A	Stored within	B	stored Not
D	body tissues	C	in body
E			
K			

→ not enough vitamin c   Radiograph 100k
  like white lines

→ in children Rickets
  in adults osteomalacia

→ inability to see in night time

→ helps form blood used in clotting

Diease of Blood

1. Anemia → low hemoglobin
   iron deficiency / hemolytic enemia (sickle cell Anemia
   erythroblastnora — RH factor mom—) child (+)
2. Polycythemia → vera (primary) increase WBC's
   (secondary) thins blood
3. Leukemia WBC.
   cancer of bone marrow   Myelocytic — acute
   ↑ granulocytes   More common in adults
   ↓ WBC
   — lymphatic — ↑ lymphocytes
   utic   ↓ lythrodes ⇒
   — acute — abrupt onset ↑ rapidly
4. Infectious Mononucleosis — kissing diease (viral) ↑WBC have antibodies
   for virus.
5. Hemophlia — inherited recessive gene found in males
6. Purpura — thrombocytopenia — little hemorages under skin, decrease in platelets

Rationale

Although the endocrine system itself cannot be imaged through diagnostic radiographs, the technologist must be aware of the disorders that are caused by abnormalities of the endocrine system. The subspecialties of radiography (nuclear medicine, CT, and MRI) are more informative in diagnosing the actual endocrine gland disorders. The radiographer, however, should remember that pathologic fractures can and do occur with many endocrine-related disorders. Therefore, patients with such disorders must be treated with extreme care so as not to aggravate their condition.

Objectives

1. (   ) Name the glands of the endocrine system.

2. (   ) Describe the functions of the anterior and posterior lobes of the pituitary gland.

3. (   ) Explain the difference between gigantism and acromegaly.

4. (   ) Explain the difference between diabetes insipidus and diabetes mellitus.

5. (   ) Describe cretinism and myxedema.

6. (   ) Name the manifestations of Graves disease.

7. (   ) Describe Cushing syndrome and Addison disease.

8. (   ) Define pheochromocytoma.

9. (   ) Explain neuroblastomas.

EXERCISE XI-1

Complete the blanks in the following statements.

1. The release of glucagon into the body is the responsibility of what organ?

   Pancreas

2. Another name for adrenaline is _norepinephrin (fight or flight)_

3. Name two manifestations of Cushing syndrome.

   moon shape face   _hirtusion_
   Sexual impotence   _hypertension_

4. What gland controls the pituitary gland?

hypothalamus

5. Name the gland that is located anteriorly in the neck.

thyroid

6. Name the two parts of the parathyroid glands.

Superior   _inferior_

7. What are the two functions of the parathyroid glands?

reduce calcium in bones
promotes calcium content in blood
regulate phosphorus

8. Name the master gland of the body. _pituatary_

9. What is the name of the funnel-shaped passage that connects the hypothalamus to the pituitary gland?

pituatary stalk

10. What are the names of the lobes of the pituitary gland?

anterior   _posterior_

11. Which lobe of the pituitary gland secretes an antidiuretic hormone that stimulates water reabsorption by tubules of the kidneys?

posterior

12. Which part of the adrenal gland is indispensable to life?

cortex

13. Which part of the adrenal gland secretes epinephrine and norepinephrine?

medulla

14. What is probably the best imaging modality to demonstrate the adrenal glands? _high resolution CT_

15. Secretion of hormones is controlled by what type of mechanism?

feedback

16. Name the two types of iodine-laden hormones.

thyroxine   _triiodothyroxine_

17. Name the male hormone secreted by the adrenal cortex.

androgen

18. Pituitary insufficiency in children causes what condition?

dwarfism

19. Premature senility (progeria) is known as

Simmond _____ syndrome.

20. Thyroid insufficiency in adults causes edema of the face and eyelids. This condition is known as _myxedema_ .

myxedema

EXERCISE XI-2

Mark the following statements "T" for true or "F" for false. If it is a false statement, reword it to make it true by changing the incorrect portions.

F   *epinephron*

___F___ 1. ~~Androgen~~ is able to cause some blood vessels to dilate to provide more blood to muscles that need oxygen.

___T___ 2. A complication of Cushing syndrome is compression fracture of the vertebral bodies.

wilms

___F___ 3. ~~Neuroblastoma~~ is the most common malignancy found in children.

___T___ 4. Diabetes mellitus results if the pancreas does not secrete insulin.

___F___ 5. A goiter is the result of enlargement of the ~~para~~thyroid gland.

___T___ 6. Dietary deficiency of iodine may cause hypothyroidism.

___T___ 7. Hyperthyroidism can produce weight loss and restlessness.

___T___ 8. Metabolism of proteins and fats is regulated by thyroid-stimulating hormone.

___T___ 9. The patient with Cushing syndrome may present with nephrocalcinosis.

___F___ 10. Spontaneous fractures caused by diffuse osteoporosis is a complication of ~~Addison disease~~.

Cushing Disease

___T___ 11. The characteristic "rugger jersey" spine is seen in patients with hyperparathyroidism as a result of renal failure.

___T___ 12. Calcification is a common finding in a neuroblastoma.

___T___ 13. Thyroid adenomas are a benign condition.

Wilms tumor

___F___ 14. A ~~neuroblastoma~~ displaces the collecting system within the kidney.

      ↳ *displaces whole kidney*

___T___ 15. Polyuria is the most common characteristic of diabetes mellitus.

___T___ 16. All of the hormones secreted by the adrenal cortex are steroids.

are suspected

___F___ 17. Patients that fall into the category of prediabetics ~~have developed~~ abnormal ~~glucose tolerance test results.~~

diabetes category

EXERCISE XI-3

Circle the letter in front of the correct answer.

1. Which of the following secretes glucocorticoids?
   A. adrenals
   B. pituitary
   C. pancreas
   D. thyroid

2. Which is a leading cause of death in persons with diabetes?
   A. arteriosclerosis
   B. gangrene
   C. hypoglycemia
   D. renal failure

3. Which is caused by pathology of the pancreas?
   A. diabetes insipidus
   B. diabetes mellitus
   C. myxedema
   D. dwarfism

4. Endocrine glands are also called
   A. salivary glands
   B. reproductive glands
   C. ductless glands
   D. sebaceous glands

5. Exophthalmos refers to a visible abnormality of the
   A. skin
   B. nose
   C. ears
   D. eyes

6. A cretin is an
   A. adult with an overactive thyroid gland
   B. adult with an underactive thyroid gland
   C. infant with an overactive thyroid gland
   D. infant with an underactive thyroid gland

7. The coloration of the skin is due to the presence of
   A. thyroid-stimulating hormone
   B. adrenaline
   C. prolactin
   D. melanin

8. The parathyroid glands secrete a hormone that regulates the metabolism of
   A. sodium
   B. calcium
   C. potassium
   D. iron

9. The thymus
   A. is found in the neck
   B. has no function
   C. produces thyroxine
   D. becomes smaller in the adult

10. Which is *not* secreted by the gonads?
    A. testosterone
    B. melatonin
    C. estrogen
    D. progesterone

11. Which hormone suppresses the amount of urine formed by promoting water reabsorption?
    A. antidiuretic hormone
    B. renin
    C. thyroid-stimulating hormone
    D. secretin

12. The thyroid function is best demonstrated by
    A. ultrasound
    B. CT
    C. MRI
    D. nuclear medicine

13. A major complication of diabetes is
    A. arteriosclerosis
    B. kidney stones
    C. pancreatic carcinoma
    D. decreased liver function

14. Functions of the parathyroid glands are to
    (1) regulate phosphorus content in blood   (2) promote calcium concentration in blood   (3) reduce calcium concentration in bones
    A. 1 and 2 only
    B. 1 and 3 only
    C. 2 and 3 only
    D. 1, 2, and 3

15. Chronic adrenocortical insufficiency is the cause of
    A. Paget disease
    B. uremia
    C. Addison disease
    D. Cushing syndrome

16. Which of the following specialties will *not* be able to visualize the pineal gland?
    A. ultrasonography
    B. CT
    C. MRI
    D. nuclear medicine

17. Which hormone is *not* secreted by the anterior lobe of the pituitary gland?
    A. somatotropin
    B. prolactin
    C. oxytocin
    D. follicle-stimulating hormone

EXERCISE XI-4

Match each of the following with the correct definition by placing the letter of the answer in the space provided. Each question has only one correct answer.

A. pituitary   E. Addison disease

B. pancreas   F. diabetes insipidus

C. adrenals   G. cretinism

D. thyroid   H. acromegaly

1. _A_ growth hormone *pituitary*

2. _C_ epinephrine *adrenals*

3. _A_ prolactin *pituitary*

4. _B_ insulin *pancreas*

5. _C_ mineralocorticoids *adrenals*

6. _A_ luteinizing hormone *pituitary*

7. _C_ glucocorticoids *adrenals*

8. _B_ glucagon *pancreas*

9. _D_ calcitonin *thyroid*

10. _A_ oxytocin *pituitary*

11. _C_ androgen *adrenals*

12. _C_ steroids *adrenals*

13. _C_ estrogen *adrenals*

14. _A_ ACTH *pituitary*

15. _A_ somatotropin *pituitary*

16. _E_ deficient amounts of glucocorticoids *addison disease*

17. _H_ enlargement of hands and feet *acromegaly*

18. _G_ insufficiency of thyroid hormone *cretinism*

19. _E_ ACTH deficiency *addison disease*

20. _F_ insufficiency of the antidiuretic hormone *diabetes insipidus*

CHAPTER XI SELF-TEST

There are 50 possible points on this self-test. Score it against the answers found in the exercises. A score of 47 points or higher indicates mastery and retention of this material.

Complete the blanks in the following statements.

1. What gland controls the pituitary gland?

   hypothalamus

2. What are the two functions of the parathyroid glands?

   reduce calcium in blood

   promotes calcium content in blood

3. Which lobe of the pituitary gland secretes an antidiuretic hormone that stimulates water reabsorption by tubules of the kidneys?

   posterior

4. Name the male hormone secreted by the adrenal cortex.

   androgen

5. Name the master gland of the body.

   pituitary gland

6. What is probably the best imaging modality to demonstrate the adrenal glands? _high resolution (CT)_

7. Premature senility (progeria) is known as

   Simmend _____ syndrome.

8. The release of glucagon into the body is the responsibility of what organ?

pancreas

9. Secretion of hormones is controlled by what type of mechanism?

feedback

10. Name two manifestations of Cushing syndrome.

~~moon~~ _shape face_   _sexual impotence_

11. What is the name of the funnel-shaped passage that connects the hypothalamus to the pituitary gland?

pituitary stalk

12. Pituitary insufficiency in children causes what condition?

Dwarfism

13. Which part of the adrenal gland is indispensable to life?

Cortex

14. Thyroid insufficiency in adults causes edema of the face and eyelids. This condition is known as _myexdema_ .

Mark the following statements "T" for true or "F" for false.

___T___ 15. Hyperthyroidism can produce weight loss and restlessness.

___T___ 16. The characteristic "rugger jersey" spine is seen in patients with hyperparathyroidism as a result of renal failure.

Epinephrone
___F___ 17. ~~Androgen~~ is able to cause some blood vessels to dilate to provide more blood to muscles that need oxygen.

Epinephrine

_F_ 18. A goiter is the result of enlargement of the ~~para~~thyroid gland.

_T_ 19. The patient with Cushing syndrome may present with nephrocalcinosis.

_F_ Wilms Tumor
20. Neuroblastoma is the most common malignancy found in children.

_T_ 21. Polyuria is the most common characteristic of diabetes mellitus.

_F_ are suspected
22. Patients that fall into the category of prediabetics ~~have developed abnor-~~
mal glucose tolerance test results.   diabetis category

_T_ 23. Calcification is a common finding in a neuroblastoma.

_F_ Wilms Tumor
24. A ~~neuroblastoma~~ will displace the collecting system within the kidney.

_F_ 25. Spontaneous fractures caused by diffuse osteoporosis is a complication of ~~Addison~~ disease.
Cushing

_T_ 26. Thyroid adenomas are a benign condition.

Circle the letter in front of the correct answer.

27. The thymus
    A. is found in the neck
    B. has no function
    C. produces thyroxine
    (D) becomes smaller in the adult

28. Exophthalmos refers to a visible abnormality of the
    A. skin
    B. nose
    C. ears
    (D) eyes

29. Which is caused by pathology of the pancreas?
    A. diabetes insipidus
    (B) diabetes mellitus
    C. myxedema
    D. dwarfism

30. The coloration of the skin is due to the presence of
    A. thyroid-stimulating hormone
    B. adrenaline
    C. prolactin
    (D) melanin

31. Which is a leading cause of death in persons with diabetes?
    A. arteriosclerosis
    B. gangrene
    C. hypoglycemia
    (D) renal failure

32. Which is not secreted by the gonads?
    A. testosterone
    B. melatonin
    C. estrogen
    D. progesterone

33. A cretin is an
    A. adult with an overactive thyroid gland
    B. adult with an underactive thyroid gland
    C. infant with an overactive thyroid gland
    D. infant with an underactive thyroid gland

34. Endocrine glands are also called
    A. salivary glands
    B. reproductive glands
    C. ductless glands
    D. sebaceous glands

35. Chronic adrenocortical insufficiency is the cause of
    A. Paget disease
    B. uremia
    C. Addison disease
    D. Cushing syndrome

36. Which hormone is *not* secreted by the anterior lobe of the pituitary gland?
    A. somatotropin
    B. prolactin
    C. oxytocin
    D. follicle-stimulating hormone

37. A major complication of diabetes is
    A. arteriosclerosis
    B. kidney stones
    C. pancreatic carcinoma
    D. decreased liver function

38. The thyroid function is best demonstrated by
    A. ultrasound
    B. CT
    C. MRI
    D. nuclear medicine

Match each of the following with the correct definition by placing the letter of the answer in the space provided. Each question has only one correct answer.

A. pituitary

B. pancreas

C. adrenals

D. thyroid

E. Addison disease

F. diabetes insipidus

G. cretinism

H. acromegaly

39. __A__ growth hormone
pituitary

40. __C__ steroids *adrenals*

41. __D__ insufficiency of thyroid hormone
thyroid

42. __F__ insufficiency of the antidiuretic hormone
diabetis insipidus

43. __A__ prolactin
pituitary

44. __B__ calcitonin
thyroid

45. __A__ luteinizing hormone
pituitary

46. __A__ somatotropin *pituitary*

47. __H__ enlargement of hands and feet *acromegaly*

48. __A__ oxytocin *pituitary*

49. __C__ mineralocorticoids *adrenals*

50. __B__ insulin *pancreas*

ANSWERS TO EXERCISES

Exercise I-1

1. symptoms, signs
2. procedure, test
3. lesions
4. manifestations, procedures
5. mortality
6. degeneration
7. trauma
8. vascular
9. red skin, heat, swelling, pain
10. alteration in vascularity, leukocytes go to area, phagocytosis, repair
11. epithelial, connective, muscle, nerve
12. voluntary, involuntary, cardiac
13. regeneration, granulation tissue
14. neoplasm, hyperplasia

Exercise I-2

1. T
2. F   a barium enema is a procedure
3. T
4. T
5. F   two disease classifications are structural and functional
6. F   allergies are structural
7. T
8. T
9. F   congestion is due to increased blood supply at the site of injury
10. F   most desirable is regeneration
11. T
12. F   linings are epithelial tissue
13. T
14. F   external agents are physical and chemical
15. F   these are tests

Exercise I-3

1. A	5. D	9. B	13. A
2. C	6. D	10. C	
3. B	7. A	11. A	
4. A	8. A	12. C	

Exercise I-4

1. Y	11. T	21. H	31. V
2. P	12. C	22. B	32. DD
3. N	13. J	23. L	33. X
4. S	14. D	24. I	
5. G	15. Q	25. W	
6. U	16. E	26. K	
7. O	17. R	27. FF	
8. M	18. CC	28. BB	
9. F	19. EE	29. Z	
10. AA	20. A	30. GG	

Exercise II-1

1. vasovagal (vagal)
2. Benadryl
3. air, oxygen, carbon dioxide, nitrous oxide
4. air, oxygen
5. gas emboli
6. barium
7. availability, atomic number, exchangeability with other ions
8. increases, high
9. low, decrease
10. allergic history
11. density
12. minor
13. BUN or creatinine, serum bilirubin
14. nonionic, ionic, monoacid, nonionic
15. 3, 2
16. carboxyl
17. viscosity, miscibility, toxicity, osmolality, persistence, type of ionic salt, iodine content
18. 300

Exercise II-2

1. T
2. T
3. F   nuclear medicine uses nuclides
4. T
5. F   radiopaques are positive media
6. T
7. T
8. T
9. F   positive media are excreted by liver or kidneys
10. T
11. F   always use low toxic media
12. F   Ethiodol is oily and does not mix
13. T
14. F   Telepaque can be used for gallbladder examinations
15. T
16. T
17. F   fast injections can cause reactions
18. F   Solu-Cortef is used in cardiac arrest cases
19. T
20. T
21. F   positive media are composed of anion and cation
22. F   iodine content is lower with meglumine salt
23. T
24. T
25. F   never use barium when a fistula exists
26. T
27. T
28. T

Exercise II-3

1. B	3. D	5. B	7. C
2. C	4. C	6. D	8. C

9. D   11. A   13. A
10. A   12. D   14. B

Exercise II-4

1. A   5. B   9. A
2. B   6. B   10. A
3. B   7. B   11. B
4. A   8. A   12. A

Exercise II-5

Table II–1.
Examinations of Systems

	Biliary	Gastrointestinal	Respiratory	Urinary	Reproductive	Neurogenic
Salpix					X	
Hypaque	X	X		X		
Gastrografin		X				
Cholegrafin	X					
Isovue	X			X		X
Conray	X			X		
Renografin	X			X		
Telepaque	X					
Lipiodol					X	
Oragrafin	X					
Sinografin					X	
Ethiodol					X	
Omnipaque				X	X	X
Dionosil			X			

Exercise III-1

1. fatigue
2. gout
3. marrow cavity
4. movement, protection, support, storage, production of red blood cells
5. transitional
6. avulsion
7. diaphysis
8. gliding, hinge, condylar, saddle, pivot, ball and socket
9. osteoclasts
10. appendicular, axial
11. positive
12. nuclear medicine, 50 percent

13. osteoclastomas
14. paraplegia, multiple myeloma
15. torus

Exercise III-2

1. F   this occurs in red bone marrow
2. T
3. T
4. F   red bone marrow is found in spongy bones
5. T
6. F   osteoblasts form bone matrix
7. T
8. T
9. F   arthrograms demonstrate all these
10. T
11. T
12. F   renal osteodystrophy and brown tumors are related
13. F   sequestrum is dead bone
14. F   metastatic tumors are far more common
15. T

Exercise III-3

1. B	11. B	21. C
2. D	12. A	22. D
3. A	13. C	23. C
4. D	14. A	24. A
5. B	15. B	25. B
6. A	16. D	26. B
7. D	17. C	27. D
8. A	18. C	28. B
9. B	19. D	29. B
10. B	20. D	30. A

Exercise III-4

1. U	11. G	21. F
2. P	12. N	22. G
3. X	13. H	23. J
4. M	14. C	24. I
5. N	15. F	25. B
6. A	16. L	26. K
7. Z	17. E	27. T
8. D	18. E	28. W
9. S	19. O	29. Q
10. I	20. X	

Exercise IV-1

1. enzymatic necrosis
2. CT
3. cholelithiasis
4. cholecystitis
5. cholangitis
6. obstructive (surgical)

7. cholesterol
8. approximately 30 minutes
9. cholecystokinin
10. calcium
11. SGOT, SGPT, alkaline phosphatase, serum bilirubin
12. alcoholism
13. cholecystectomy
14. CT, PTC, T-tube cholangiography, HIDA and PIPIDA nuclear medicine scans, ultrasonography
15. hepatitis A
16. porcelain gallbladder
17. pancreatitis
18. ultrasonography
19. blockage of the cystic duct, hepatitis, blockage of hepatic ducts
20. acinar cells, beta cells, isle of Langerhans
21. water (97%)
22. to concentrate the bile in the tube to prevent air accumulation
23. poor patient preparation
24. a. left lobe of liver
    b. quadrate lobe
    c. caudate lobe
    d. right lobe of liver
    e. Reidel's lobe of liver
    f. portal vein
    g. IVC
    h. falciform ligament

Exercise IV-2

1. T
2. F   nutrients go the liver via the portal vein
3. F   this exam is a PTC
4. F   biliary system includes the gallbladder, liver, and bile ducts
5. T
6. F   it is caused by cirrhosis
7. T
8. F   Cholegrafin was used for an IVC. Contrasts such as Renografin, Conray, or Isovue are used for a T-tube cholangiogram
9. T
10. F   by nuclear medicine
11. F   it is located at the cystic duct
12. T
13. T
14. T
15. F   the liver produces bile
16. F   it is a study of the gallbladder and bile ducts
17. F   detoxification takes place in the liver
18. T
19. F   best demonstrated by CT and angiography
20. F   adenocarcinomas are most common
21. T
22. T
23. T
24. T   but only as an incidental finding
25. F   remain NPO for approximately 10 hours

Exercise IV-3

1. B	11. C
2. C	12. D
3. A	13. D
4. C	14. A
5. B	15. D
6. D	16. C
7. C	17. D
8. A	18. B
9. B	19. D
10. B	20. B

Exercise IV-4

1. F	11. B
2. D	12. K
3. I	13. H
4. A	14. D
5. B	15. G
6. G	16. J
7. C	17. N
8. A	18. F
9. I	19. L
10. M	20. A

Exercise V-1

1. shelving
2. Meckel diverticulum
3. dysphagia
4. porcelain gallbladder
5. ileum
6. volvulus
7. rectal columns
8. adult
9. pulsion; traction
10. cathartic colon
11. Barrett esophagus
12. cecum, colon, rectum
13. lesser curvature
14. phytobezoar, trichobezoar
15. Valsalva
16. small bowel
17. taenia coli
18. hypotonic duodenography
19. percutaneous transluminal angioplasty
20. may perforate the esophagus and cause an abscess
21. greater curvature
22. duodenal
23. imperforate anus; rectal atresia
24. small bowel
25. fistula

Exercise V-2

1. T
2. T
3. F   Meckel diverticulum is found in the ileum
4. T
5. F   Ligament of Trietz demarcates the junction
6. T
7. F   Esophageal rupture is due to violent vomiting
8. F   Zenker is a pulsion tick
9. T
10. F   Prolapse occurs at the pyloric channel
11. F   Greatest amount of digestion occurs in the small bowel
12. F   This patient should be tested for esophageal carcinoma
13. T
14. T
15. F   Shelving is demonstrated in esophageal carcinoma
16. T
17. F   This is a rolling, or paraesophageal, hernia
18. T
19. F   Traction diverticula are triangular
20. T

Exercise V-3

1. C	6. C	11. B
2. C	7. C	12. A
3. C	8. A	13. B
4. C	9. C	14. D
5. A	10. A	15. C

Exercise V-4

1. R	8. P	15. F	22. E
2. N	9. C	16. U	23. T
3. O	10. A	17. S	24. R
4. J	11. B	18. F	25. A
5. I	12. R	19. P	
6. A	13. P	20. P	
7. K	14. P	21. B	

Drawings

1. N	12. L
2. A	13. F
3. J	14. B
4. K	15. R
5. C	16. S
6. U	17. E
7. Q	18. D
8. V	19. O
9. I	20. G
10. M	21. H
11. P	22. T

Exercise VI-1

1. incompetent ureteral valve
2. trigone
3. BUN, creatinine
4. pancreas, duodenum, right adrenal
5. nephron
6. produce urine, secrete urine, regulate fluid in the blood, regulate electrolytes
7. bead-chain cystogram
8. renin
9. hypertensive intravenous pyelogram
10. renal agenesis
11. horseshoe
12. renal artery, renal vein, nerves, lymph tissue, and renal pelvis
13. pyelitis
14. duplication
15. polycystic renal disease

Exercise VI-2

1. F   Intravenous pyelograms are done to locate masses, abnormal laboratory values, calculi
2. T
3. F   The medulla consists of the pyramids, tubules, and papillae
4. T
5. F   Fluoroscopy is used to position the patient
6. T
7. T
8. T
9. F   Nephron is found in the cortex
10. T
11. T
12. F   Ureteroceles are found in the bladder
13. T
14. F   BUN is the most important laboratory test
15. T

Exercise VI-3

1. A	6. C	11. A
2. B	7. A	12. C
3. C	8. D	13. C
4. B	9. A	14. B
5. C	10. B	15. C

Exercise VI-4

Pathology

1. D	11. A
2. K	12. J
3. F	13. A
4. C	14. L
5. H	15. A
6. B	16. D
7. J	17. E
8. F	18. H
9. A	19. B
10. I	20. E

Special Procedures

1.	D	6.	E	11.	F
2.	A	7.	G	12.	L
3.	B	8.	I	13.	H
4.	K	9.	E	14.	B
5.	J	10.	L	15.	C

Exercise VII-1

1. fundus, body, cervix
2. anteverted, anteflexed
3. fornix
4. uterus, ovaries, uterine tube, vagina
5. breast
6. spermatocele
7. cervical
8. lobule
9. Cowper (bulbourethral)
10. proliferative, secretory, menstrual
11. involution
12. spermatogenesis
13. testosterone
14. produces pain
15. craniocaudal, mediolateral oblique
16. prevents scatters, helps with compression, makes positioning easier
17. müllerian ducts
18. septate
19. A. vagina   F. body
    B. fornix   G. ovary
    C. external os   H. fundus
    D. cervix   I. uterine tube
    E. internal os   J. fimbriated extremity
20. A. retroversion
    B. anteflexion
    C. retroflexion

Exercise VII-2

1. F pyosalpinx may result if PID goes untreated
2. T
3. T
4. T
5. F adenomyosis coexists with endometriosis
6. F PID is caused by veneral disease in 50–60% of cases
7. T
8. F endometrial carcinoma shows indented bladder
9. T
10. T
11. F young women have dense breasts
12. F malignant tumors show calcifications
13. F mammographic units have molybdenum targets
14. F endometriosis is the growth of tissue outside the uterus
15. T
16. T
17. F undescended testis is cryptorchidism
18. T

19. T
20. T

Exercise VII-3

1. C	6. A	11. B
2. C	7. D	12. C
3. A	8. A	13. B
4. A	9. B	14. D
5. D	10. C	15. C

Exercise VII-4

1. C	11. F
2. K	12. O
3. K	13. N
4. G	14. P
5. H	15. Q
6. D	16. S
7. J	17. M
8. L	18. O
9. F	19. C
10. G	20. B

Drawing

21. C	25. A
22. E	26. F
23. D	27. G
24. B	

Exercise VIII-1

1. larynx
2. carina
3. left
4. oblique (major)
5. congestive heart failure
6. aqueous, oily
7. catheter insertion, percutaneous transtracheal, aspiration
8. hilum
9. abscess
10. visceral, parietal
11. bronchography
12. silicosis, asbestosis, berylliosis
13. cystic fibrosis
14. alveoli
15. superior, anterior, middle, posterior
16. pulmonary embolism
17. air bronchogram
18. pneumothorax
19. bronchiectasis
20. atelectasis

Exercise VIII-2

1. T
2. F   emphysema and COPD are interchangeable names

3. T
4. T
5. F   causes the appearance of congestive heart failure, magnification
6. T
7. T
8. F   should take single exposure films of expiration and inspiration
9. T
10. F   bronchitis is inflammation of the bronchi
11. T
12. T
13. T
14. T
15. T
16. F   pneumonia is inflammation of the lungs
17. T
18. T
19. T
20. F   heart magnification appears greater on the AP radiograph

Exercise VIII-3

1. D	7. A	13. C
2. A	8. C	14. D
3. A	9. C	15. B
4. A	10. D	16. C
5. B	11. C	17. D
6. B	12. D	

Exercise VIII-4

1. S	11. G
2. R	12. B
3. T	13. H
4. C	14. I
5. N	15. O
6. U	16. E
7. P	17. A
8. D	18. M
9. X	19. P
10. Q	20. W

Exercise IX-1

1. A. right ventricle
   B. IVC
   C. triscuspid valve
   D. right atrium
   E. pulmonary semilunar valve
   F. right pulmonary veins
   G. right pulmonary arteries
   H. SVC
   I. left common carotid
   J. aortic arch
   K. pulmonary artery
   L. aortic semilunar valve
   M. left atrium
   N. mitral valve

O. left ventricle
P. septum
Q. endocardium
R. myocardium
S. pericardium
T. thoracic aorta
2. lymphatics
3. superficial, deep
4. saccular, dissecting, fusiform
5. A. right atrium
B. tricuspid valve
C. right ventricle
D. pulmonary valve
E. pulmonary artery
F. lung
G. pulmonary vein
H. left atrium
I. mitral valve
J. left ventricle
K. aortic valve
L. aorta
6. percutaneous transluminal angioplasty
7. ultrasonography (echocardiography)
8. tuberculosis, viral infection
9. tonsils, thymus, adenoids

Exercise IX-2

1. F thrombus is a blood clot in any vessel
2. T
3. F myocardial infarction is an acquired diseased area of the heart wall
4. T
5. T
6. T
7. F this takes oxygenated blood to the body
8. T
9. F RAO is 45 degrees, the LAO is 60 degrees
10. F left common carotid artery branches off the arch. The right common carotid branches off the innominate artery
11. T
12. F left atrioventricular is bicuspid. The right valve is the tricuspid
13. F this allows blood to flow back into the left atrium
14. T
15. T
16. F lymph nodes are the filtering portion
17. T
18. T
19. F oxygenated blood goes from the left ventricle into the aorta
20. T

Exercise IX-3

1. D	6. C	11. A
2. A	7. C	12. C
3. D	8. B	13. B
4. C	9. A	14. A
5. D	10. B	15. D

16. D	21. A	26. B
17. C	22. C	27. B
18. C	23. C	28. A
19. A	24. A	29. D
20. D	25. D	30. A

Exercise IX-4

1. N	11. U
2. M	12. A
3. P	13. B
4. R	14. G
5. S	15. H
6. K	16. T
7. O	17. F
8. E	18. L
9. I	19. C
10. D	20. Q

Special Procedures

21. A	26. B
22. F	27. C
23. B	28. C
24. E	29. F
25. D	30. A

Exercise X-1

1. A. anterior horn of lateral ventricle
   B. body of lateral ventricle
   C. posterior horn of lateral ventricle
   D. inferior horn of lateral ventricle
   E. foramen of Monro
   F. third ventricle
   G. aqueduct of Sylvius
   H. posterior superior recess
   I. fourth ventricle
   J. foramen of Luschka
2. hydrocephalus
3. cisterna magna or cervical area
4. autonomic
5. central, autonomic, peripheral
6. cerebrospinal system
7. brain, spinal cord
8. neurons
9. cerebrum (forebrain), mesencephalon (midbrain), hindbrain
10. thalamus, hypothalamus, third ventricle
11. correlates optic and tactile impulses, auditory reflexes; regulation of muscle tone, body posture, and equilibrium
12. cerebrospinal fluid
13. pia mater, arachnoid, dura mater
14. pia and arachnoid meninges
15. sympathetic, parasympathetic
16. air, oxygen
17. brain may herniate toward the foramen magnum
18. ventriculoatrial, ventriculoperitoneal

19. spina bifida
20. spina bifida occulta
21. meningocele, myelocele, myelomeningocele
22. atheroma, hypertension
23. circle of Willis
24. emboli
25. subdural, epidural (extradural), subarachnoid, intracerebral (intraparen-chymal)
26. linear, comminuted, depressed
27. concussion, contusion, fracture, hemorrhage
28. osteomyelitis
29. astrocytoma
30. pituitary adenoma, craniopharyngioma
31. foraminal widening
32. halo sign

Exercise X-2

1. T
2. T
3. T
4. T
5. F   most common primary brain tumor is a glioma
6. F   most common myelography is subarachnoid
7. T
8. T
9. F   this is a meningocele
10. T

Exercise X-3

1. A	7. A	13. A
2. C	8. D	14. B
3. D	9. C	15. A
4. D	10. A	16. B
5. C	11. C	17. B
6. A	12. C	18. B

Exercise X-4

1. O	11. G
2. M	12. R
3. K	13. D
4. F	14. B
5. Q	15. E
6. C	16. S
7. J	17. I
8. N	18. H
9. F	19. A
10. P	20. T

Exercise XI-1

1. pancreas
2. norepinephrine (fight or flight)
3. moon-shaped face, hypertension, sexual impotence, hirsutism
4. hypothalamus
5. thyroid

6. superior, inferior
7. reduce calcium in bones, promote calcium content in blood, regulate phosphorus content in the blood and bones
8. pituitary
9. pituitary stalk
10. anterior, posterior
11. posterior
12. cortex
13. medulla
14. high-resolution CT
15. feedback
16. thyroxine, triiodothyronine
17. androgen
18. dwarfism
19. Simmond
20. myxedema

Exercise XI-2

1. F epinephrine
2. T
3. F Wilms tumor is the most common
4. T
5. F it is from the thyroid gland
6. T
7. T
8. T
9. T
10. F this is a complication of Cushing syndrome
11. T
12. T
13. T
14. F Wilms tumor displaces the collecting system, whereas a neuroblastoma displaces the entire kidney
15. T
16. T
17. F these patients are in the "suspected" diabetes category

Exercise XI-3

1. A	6. D	11. A	16. A
2. D	7. D	12. D	17. C
3. B	8. B	13. A	
4. C	9. D	14. D	
5. D	10. B	15. C	

Exercise XI-4

1. A	6. A	11. C	16. E
2. C	7. C	12. C	17. H
3. A	8. B	13. C	18. G
4. B	9. D	14. A	19. E
5. C	10. A	15. A	20. F